YOUR FERTILITY SIGNALS

Everyone knows that tears signal sadness, and sweat shows that the body is warm. Just as naturally, a woman's slippery cervical mucus signals when she can get pregnant.

Reading your body's simple fertility signals takes just moments a day. And by using the signals, you can enhance body awareness, lovingly conceive your children, or avoid conception naturally as you choose.

What they're saying about YOUR FERTILITY SIGNALS...

BOOKLIST
"...one of the most straightforward self-help books on fertility...does much to dispel the mystery and imagined difficulty of 'natural' birth control."

MOTHERING MAGAZINE
"This is the book I've been waiting to see! The most simple, comprehensive, and all-encompassing book about Fertility Awareness on the market today. It's well organized, visually beautiful and easy to comprehend."

This book is sold at independent stores as well as at major chains such as
B. Dalton, Barnes and Nobel, and Waldenbooks. You might want to phone first to make
sure a copy is on hand or can be ordered. You may also order directly from the publisher,
using the coupon at the back of the book.

Please tell your bookseller, librarian, and natural food store owner
they may order **Your Fertility Signals** from these wholesalers:

Baker & Taylor
Bookhouse
Bookpeople
Brodart
Emery Pratt

Ingram
Midwest Library Service
New Leaf
Nutri-Books

Your Fertility Signals is available in English, Spanish, German, Chinese directly from Smooth
Stone Press. In South and Central America, obtain **Sus signos de fertilidad** from grupo
editorial norma, (ISBN 958-04-2946-4). In Europe, **Signale der Fruchtbarkeit**, is available from
Martin Ehrenwirth Verlag, (ISBN 3-431-03317-2). In Taiwan, the **Chinese version** is available
from Morning Star Publishers (TAIYA, ISBN 957-9643-27-X).

CATALOGING DATA

613.9'434
Win

Winstein, Merryl

Your fertility signals, using them to achieve or avoid pregnancy naturally.
Includes index, references, glossary. Fully illustrated.

1. Birth control/contraception - natural, popular works. 2. Fertility awareness.
3. Infertility - overcoming naturally. 4. Ovulation/mucus method.
5. Temperature method. 6. "Rhythm" method, alternatives to. I. Author. II. Title.

LIBRARY OF CONGRESS CATALOG CARD NUMBER 87-92011

ISBN: Paperback only, 0-9619401-0-7 $13.95 USA

Printed in USA, January 1999

Also from Smooth Stone Press, two young girl's novels by Iyotsna Sreenivasan:
The Moon Over Crete, illustrated by Sim Gellman
Aruna's Journeys, illustrated by Merryl Winstein
and
Bread, Soups & Salads, a cookbook by Sharon Winstein

YOUR FERTILITY SIGNALS

Using Them to

Achieve or Avoid Pregnancy

Naturally

by

MERRYL WINSTEIN

Smooth Stone Press

P.O. Box 19875
St. Louis, Missouri 63144 U.S.A.

IMPORTANT MESSAGE TO THE READER

I have written this book in order to make it easy for you to understand and use your fertility signals. But I'd like to emphasize that this is an educational book, NOT a medical book. Whenever you have a health problem or question, be sure to see your health practitioner.

*I want you to be aware that just like the Pill, diaphragm, I.U.D. or condom, natural fertility control is not foolproof. **The possibility of pregnancy does exist no matter how diligently you may follow the guidelines for naturally avoiding pregnancy.** However, the more carefully you follow the directions, the more likely it is that you will achieve the results you desire.*

The only form of birth control which is 100% effective is complete avoidance of sexual relations.

*Many authorities advise using condoms with spermicides in an attempt to avoid catching or spreading AIDS or other sexually transmitted diseases. But please understand...**natural fertility control is NOT a method of preventing the spread of AIDS.** And this book is not about AIDS prevention. This book merely explains how to achieve or avoid **pregnancy** without the need for contraceptives.*

Avoiding pregnancy naturally requires frequent daily observations of the fertility signals, keeping a daily chart, and cooperation of both partners. This method puts YOU in charge of your fertility. It's simple and you can do it!

Sincerely,
Merryl Winstein

Acknowledgements

*I extend my deepest gratitude to **Drs. John and Evelyn Billings**, who developed the modern, simplified © Billings Ovulation Method, and who have devoted their lives to promoting and teaching it throughout the world.*

I am also profoundly indebted to the following people whose generosity and friendship helped make this book a reality. Thanks to...

***Bob Borcherding**, for allowing me to use his computer and computer expertise without limit; **Suzannah Cooper**, of Fertility Awareness Services, who enthusiastically pored over nearly every draft of the manuscript in progress, and shared her fertility awareness library; **Mary Shivanandan**, of KM Associates, for her encouragement, networking contacts, and editorial insights; **Dr. Evelyn Billings**, for her thorough and candid commentary; **Barbara Feldman**, of the Fertility Awareness Center, for her pointed and observant opinions and corrections; and **Sara Rose**, of Alabama Fertility Awareness Services, and **Louise Smith** for their invaluable input. Of course I must thank the many readers who have corresponded with me, learned fertility awareness from the book, and asked the questions I've attempted to answer in this edition.*

*The physical beauty of this book owes much to the efforts of **Paul Johnson**, **Dave Runyon** and **Lauren Cunningham** at Paragon Typographers, who expertly set the type. Also, to **Les Rothweil**, **Rosanna Cerutti**, and the staff of Artcraft Graphic Services, who created superb color separations for the cover.*

*Last but not least, I wish to thank my mother, **Sharon Winstein**, for teaching me to trust the powers of my own body, and my brother, **Mark Winstein**, for sharing his excitement and business acumen. Most of all, I extend my appreciation to my loving husband, **Richard Hibbs**, who encouraged and supported me, and always believed in the importance of this book.*

Contents

YOUR FERTILITY SIGNALS
The Facts

The fertile phase is just a few days

A woman is potentially fertile for only a few days during each menstrual cycle. This means from the beginning of menstruation, to the day before her next period, there are only a handful of days during which lovemaking may result in pregnancy. The rest of the days are infertile, and nothing can cause a pregnancy then.

Fertility signals are easy to recognize

Using the first few chapters of this book as a guide, a woman will find she can easily identify her infertile and fertile days. All she needs to do is watch for the natural signs her body provides. Observing the signals takes about a minute per day, and learning to use them takes only one or two cycles.

What are the signals?

The three major fertility signals are changes in a woman's

- *CERVICAL MUCUS*
- *BASAL BODY TEMPERATURE*
- *CERVIX POSITION AND SHAPE*

CERVICAL MUCUS — the most important sign

The cervix is the "gateway" between the uterus and vagina. It produces wet, slippery mucus, which signals fertility. You may have already noticed your own wet fertile mucus in the past. Women in every culture around the world have slippery mucus during the fertile phase.

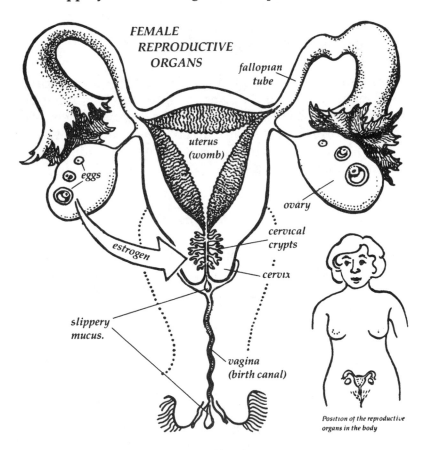

FEMALE REPRODUCTIVE ORGANS

fallopian tube

uterus (womb)

eggs

ovary

estrogen

cervical crypts

cervix

slippery mucus.

vagina (birth canal)

Position of the reproductive organs in the body

Ripening eggs cause mucus production

During each cycle, 10-20 of a woman's immature eggs begin to ripen. As they develop, they secrete the hormone estrogen. Estrogen prompts the cervix to secrete wet, increasingly slippery mucus, which slides down to the vaginal opening.

Mucus signals fertility in all types of cycles

Whether your cycles are long, short, regular or irregular, **slippery mucus signals that eggs are developing and you are fertile**. Mucus announces that one of the eggs will soon *ovulate*, or burst out of the ovary, ready for fertilization.

Ovulation ⸗ release of the live egg

One egg (or two for fraternal twins) finally bursts out of the ovary. Eighty-five percent of the time, ovulation takes place on the last mucus day or the day after.[1] About 10-15% of the time, ovulation may happen up to two or three days before or after the last mucus day.[2,3]

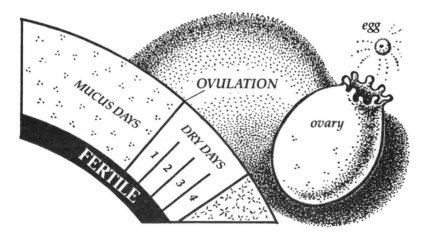

When is a woman fertile?

After ovulating, the egg lives and can be fertilized for 12-24 hours. But since mucus may keep the man's sperm cells alive until ovulation, **a woman is considered fertile on any day of mucus, plus the first four dry days in a row after the mucus ends**.

Conception of a baby

Conception takes place when the woman's ovulated egg unites with one tiny sperm cell from the man. The egg and sperm meet inside the woman's fallopian tube.

Mucus nourishes the man's sperm until ovulation

Normally, natural acids in the vagina will kill sperm cells within a matter of hours. But mucus keeps sperm cells alive.

Suppose you have some slippery mucus on Monday morning, and you make love that evening. The mucus will nourish and protect the man's sperm cells for three to five days inside the cervix.

When you finally ovulate, perhaps on Thursday or Friday, the waiting sperm rush up to meet and fertilize the egg, and you may become pregnant.

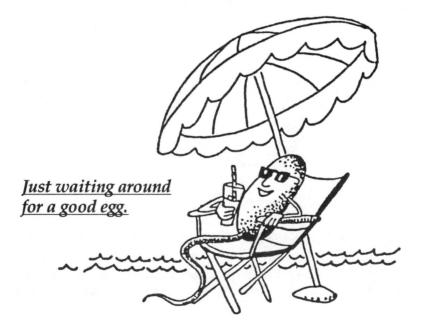

Just waiting around for a good egg.

For conception to happen, there must be mucus

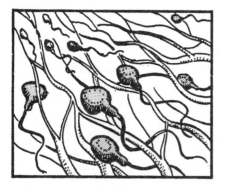

The slippery mucus is full of elongated channels or swimming lanes which permit the sperm to swim through the cervix.

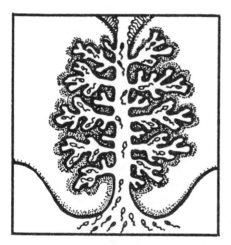

After intercourse, a man's sperm cells can wait up to five days inside tiny cave-like crypts in the cervix. There they are sheltered by the wet fertile mucus.[4]

Without enough fertile mucus, the cervix is blocked, and conception cannot happen.[5]

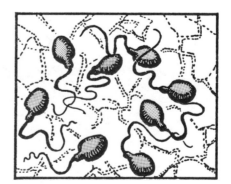

Finding and charting your own mucus

Observing your mucus is easy. Just wipe across your vaginal opening *before and after* each use of the toilet. Only a few seconds are required at each bathroom visit, so accurately observing your mucus takes only a minute or so per day.

You'll learn more about checking the mucus on pages 22-25. After writing down your mucus observations before bedtime, you'll soon have a chart which resembles this one.

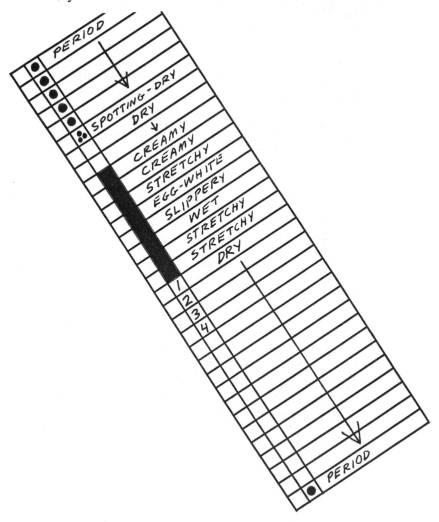

How long is the fertile phase?

The length of the fertile phase varies from cycle to cycle, but is usually about 8-14 days.

Do women ovulate during orgasm?

Orgasm does not cause ovulation in women, although it may do so in other animals such as rabbits. Women ovulate only after a complex sequence of hormonal events has taken place.

When is a man fertile?

A man is fertile all of the time after puberty (approximately age 9-13). He is always producing new sperm cells which can fertilize a woman's egg, allowing pregnancy to begin.

Using the mucus sign for natural fertility control

A woman is fertile whenever she has wet, slippery mucus and until the evening of the fourth dry day in a row afterward. During this time of shared fertility, a couple decides whether to make love and expect to become pregnant, or to avoid all genital-to-genital contact (including early withdrawal) in order to avoid pregnancy. The choice is always theirs.

Since natural fertility control is a cooperative method, it works best in a loving relationship. Success is also greater for the woman who checks her mucus at every visit to the toilet, and firmly states that she is fertile, infertile, or temporarily unsure.

SECONDARY FERTILITY SIGNS

Temperature shows when ovulation is over

Changes in your daily temperature (basal body temperature) show when ovulation is finished and you are no longer fertile. Temperature method directions begin on page 46.

The temperature chart, along with the mucus chart, may help show whether a woman ovulates before, during, or after the last day of mucus. Accordingly, couples may choose their most fertile time for conception.[6]

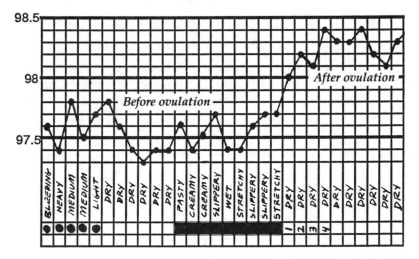

One woman's temperature chart

Cervix position and shape

If you gently touch the cervix with your fingers once a day you'll notice how the cervix changes throughout the cycle. A firm, pointed shape generally indicates low estrogen. As estrogen and fertility increase, the cervix softens, opens up, and rises higher so that it is harder to reach. Around the time of ovulation, when estrogen levels suddenly drop, you can feel the hardened, closed cervix back in its lower position. Observing your cervix is interesting, and fairly reliable for some women, but it is *not required* for effective natural fertility control.

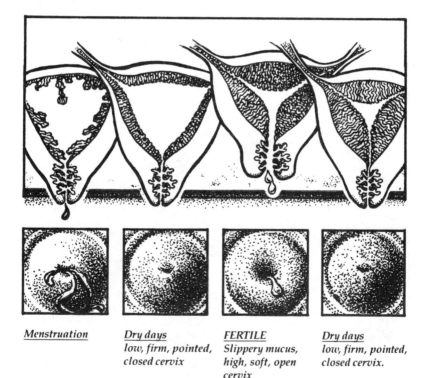

| <u>Menstruation</u> | <u>Dry days</u> *low, firm, pointed, closed cervix* | <u>FERTILE</u> *Slippery mucus, high, soft, open cervix* | <u>Dry days</u> *low, firm, pointed, closed cervix.* |

A woman is fertile on all days and nights of mucus. Fertility continues through the evening of the fourth dry day in a row after the mucus ends.

General fertility signals

Spotting and bleeding indicate possible fertility, since the hormonal changes leading to ovulation may cause spotting too.

Mittelschmertz (abdominal pain), breast tenderness, backaches, or bloating show that your reproductive hormone levels are rising and falling. However, these signs *do not* tell exactly when you can or can't get pregnant.

A mucus chart is a good place to record emotions, mood swings and energy changes. Many women's emotions are closely linked to fertility changes. Charting helps some women predict and plan for cyclic mood swings.

THE FEMALE CYCLE
OF FERTILITY AND INFERTILITY

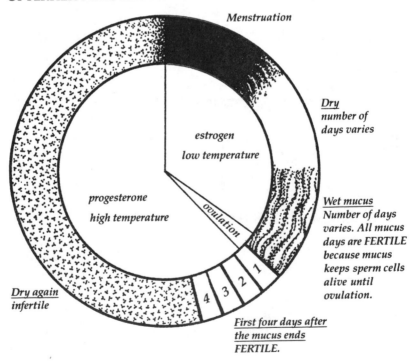

Menstruation

Dry
number of
days varies

estrogen
low temperature

progesterone
high temperature

ovulation

Wet mucus
Number of days
varies. All mucus
days are FERTILE
because mucus
keeps sperm cells
alive until
ovulation.

Dry again
infertile

First four days after
the mucus ends
FERTILE.

Which signals should you use?

You may use mucus alone, mucus plus temperature, or mucus, temperature and cervical change for fertility awareness. This book tells how to use each signal.

MUCUS tells whether you can or can't get pregnant each and every day.

TEMPERATURE shows that ovulation is finished and you are no longer fertile.

CERVICAL CHANGE indicates general changes in your estrogen level.

The signals are easy to understand

In just moments a day, your fertility signals will tell whether you can or can't get pregnant.

Let this book guide you to greater awareness of your fertility. If you wish, consult with any of the hundreds of experienced teachers who are eager to assist you.* Soon you too will experience the marvelous power of living in harmony with your fertility.

*Teachers are listed near the end of this book.

Added Dimensions

Couples who understand the fertility signals may...

- **prevent or postpone pregnancy naturally**
- **become pregnant as they desire**
- **reduce or eliminate contraceptive usage**

No matter how long, short or irregular a woman's cycles may be, the natural signs will reflect her fertility changes clearly each and every day.

The signals are accurate during any reproductive situation including breastfeeding, pre-menopause, or after stopping contraceptive pills. The signs are also accurate during times of illness or stress, for those who are willing to exercise additional patience and care.

Couples having difficulty becoming pregnant may soon learn to recognize their most fertile times. Not only that, but the fertility signals help identify many specific infertility problems.

Fertility awareness is not rhythm

Using the calendar rhythm method, women took their temperature and counted the number of days in previous cycles. Then they merely *guessed* which days might be fertile in the future. Since cycle lengths normally vary, rhythm did not always work very well. In contrast, cervical mucus *as observed by women themselves* is a scientifically verified sign that eggs are actually developing and that a woman is potentially fertile.[1] Rhythm failed, but fertility awareness works.

Added benefits of natural fertility control

- Both partners share the responsibility for preventing or achieving pregnancy.

- The couple enjoys a wonderful sense of fun, freedom and security once they know just when they can or can't get pregnant.

- Couples can avoid the interruption, mess and often harmful side effects of contraceptive devices and chemicals.

- Intimacy increases when loving and sexual feelings flow spontaneously into lovemaking.

- Fertility awareness satisfies curiosity about natural body processes. And it's free after the initial expenses of learning *(Volunteer teachers, often religious, may charge very little; paid instructors usually charge from $65-$250.)*

- Natural fertility control honors religious or personal convictions prohibiting artificial contraception.

- Charting the fertility signals can help couples predict cyclic emotional swings, and treat premenstrual discomfort.

- Understanding your normal fertility signs will help you become immediately aware of anything abnormal which may indicate infections, cysts, or other changes in your gynecological health.

- And finally, fertility awareness wonderfully enhances a woman's feelings of self-confidence and independence. At the same time it expands each partner's ability to trust, cooperate and love.

How effective is natural fertility control?

When taught and used correctly, the ovulation method (mucus only) is, biologically speaking, 97-99% effective for preventing undesired pregnancies,[2] — just as effective as the Pill, I.U.D., or diaphragm.

However, about 20 of any 100 couples who learn the ovulation method in one year do make love on fertile days, and as expected, they usually become pregnant.

The 20% figure is sometimes misconstrued as evidence that cervical mucus is not a reliable fertility signal, or that the ovulation method is too hard for women to use and understand.

The fact is that couples who make love on fertile days, or when they are unsure of their fertility, are *correctly following the ovulation method guidelines for becoming pregnant*. At all times, couples may freely choose to make love while fertile or unsure about their fertility. Naturally they should expect pregnancy to result. Couples may just as freely decide to avoid intercourse and genital contact while fertile or unsure, thereby avoiding pregnancy.

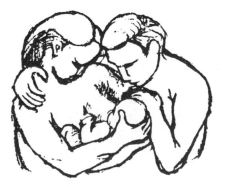

Conduct an informal survey.

How many women do you know who used contraceptives correctly and became pregnant anyway? Compare that with the numbers of women you can find who became pregnant while using natural methods *correctly* for avoiding pregnancy. In the author's experience, the possibility of a surprise pregnancy while using natural methods correctly for avoiding pregnancy is very slim. Yet the author frequently meets women whose contraceptives have allowed pregnancy to happen — statistics notwithstanding.

When do contraceptives fail?

Contraceptive failures can only happen during the woman's easily recognized fertile phase. Knowing this, couples who depend on contraceptives can and should use extra care while the woman is fertile. During the infertile phase, it is the woman's natural infertility, not the power of a contraceptive, which keeps her from getting pregnant.

Natural methods put the couple in charge

Awareness, motivation, love and cooperation are indispensable for successful long-term natural fertility control. In order to use natural methods, a woman herself must take the time to learn about her body, and watch the fertility signals each day and night. And a couple must cooperate if they are to naturally avoid pregnancy through the years.

Couples who use natural fertility control cannot blame a device or pharmaceutical company for a surprise pregnancy. They know exactly when they are fertile, infertile, or unsure of their fertility. This sense of shared responsibility appeals strongly to some women and men, and is one reason that others decide against using natural methods.

Learning

About 90% of the women in the 1978 World Health Organization's five-country study learned to recognize their mucus pattern within thirty days.[1] You can too. Directions for finding the mucus begin on page 21.

Learn quickly while avoiding intercourse for awhile

The shortest, surest way to learn the mucus signal is to watch your fertility pattern unfold while avoiding intercourse and genital-to-genital contact for three to four weeks. Why? Because slippery arousal fluid, semen, or spermicides can be as wet and slippery as the mucus you are looking for.

Pregnancy can occur when new learners assume they know which days are infertile before experiencing an entire cycle. So while learning, please be extra careful — it's no time for taking chances.

Your first chart may look something like this:

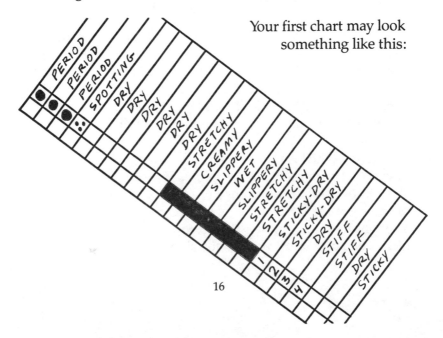

Learn more slowly while continuing to use barrier methods with spermicide

If you continue using contraceptive barriers, such as condom and foam, diaphragm and jelly, or cervical cap and cream, you can still learn about your fertility signals. Just remember that you'll be depending *entirely* on the barrier and spermicide to prevent pregnancy. You *won't be using* the ovulation method or sympto-thermal method at all.

Learning the mucus pattern will probably take about four to six months if you keep on using contraceptive barriers and slippery spermicides. The temperature signal will be apparent right away. However, you cannot learn your mucus or temperature pattern while you are still taking contraceptive Pills.

Make consistent observations; soon your awareness of the pattern will grow, and with it the confidence that you can control your fertility naturally.

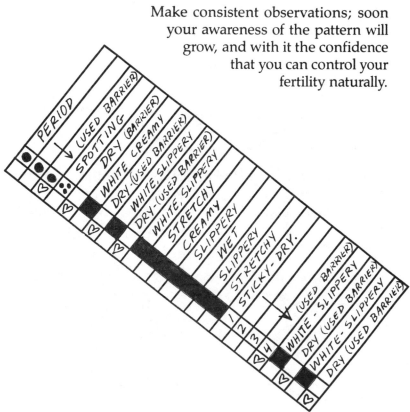

The fertile time is designed to help you become pregnant regardless of barriers

You are fertile any time you have wet, smooth, slippery, blood-tinged or stretchy mucus, and for the first four dry days in a row after the mucus or spotting ends. While fertile, or whenever you are unsure of your fertility, you are free to decide just how careful you wish to be about achieving or avoiding pregnancy. If you want to be as certain as possible of avoiding pregnancy naturally, follow these guidelines while you are fertile or unsure:

- **Refrain from** *all* **genital-to-genital contact and intercourse.**

- **Avoid intercourse even while using contraceptives.** Pregnancies do occur even while couples use contraceptives, and each pregnancy begins during the fertile time. When a barrier fails during the fertile phase, mucus does its job of naturally helping the sperm survive until ovulation.

- **Do not use "early withdrawal."** A drop of fluid filled with thousands of sperm cells is already ready and waiting long before the man ejaculates.

- **Don't transfer a drop of semen by hand or other means to the inside or the outside of the vagina.** Channels in the fertile mucus can guide the swimming sperm up through the vagina and cervix and pregnancy can begin, even if you haven't had intercourse.

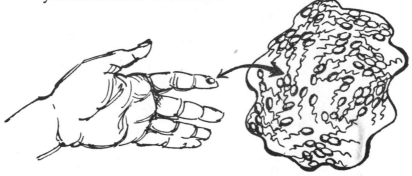

What about using barriers without slippery spermicides?

Although a condom without foam is less confusing to your mucus pattern, it will prevent pregnancy only if it stays on and if no semen leaks from it. Condoms alone are only 80% effective; about 20% of the couples using condoms alone for a year get pregnant. Similarly, a diaphragm or cervical cap without jelly or cream generally won't work.* The only purpose of these devices is to keep the jelly in place. Microscopically small sperm cells can easily swim around the plastic barriers.

Using the I.U.D. or contraceptive Pill

The I.U.D., or intrauterine device, may cause confusing mucus when the string irritates your cervical crypts. In addition, the string wicks harmful bacteria up into the uterus. The results? Painful infections of the uterus and fallopian tubes, scarring, sterility (permanent infertility), and sometimes death. Because of these serious health risks, I.U.D.'s are not recommended by most doctors.

Artificial hormones in the Pill thoroughly suppress your natural mucus and temperature signals. But as soon as you stop taking oral contraceptives, you can start learning the natural fertility patterns. In the chapter entitled *"After the Pill,"* you will read about the type of mucus pattern to expect while your body recovers from oral contraceptives.

---

*Some women prefer using a cervical cap or condom without spermicide, although either practice increases the chances of an unexpected pregnancy.

YOUR MUCUS SIGNAL
The Ovulation Method

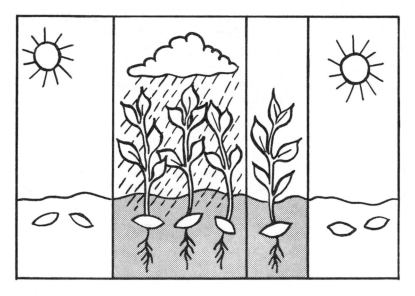

When the ground is dry, a seed cannot sprout.

When it rains, and for a few days after the rain stops, seeds can grow.

Dry again, seeds cannot grow.

Every day, the mucus tells whether you are fertile,
infertile, approaching ovulation, or finished ovulating.

You may use the mucus signal alone
to effectively achieve or avoid pregnancy.

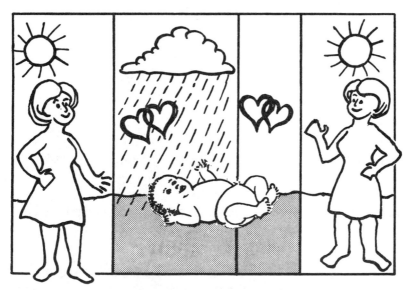

*When a
woman is dry
(no mucus),
a baby cannot
start to grow.*

*When a woman has wet
mucus, and for a few days
after the mucus ends, a
baby can be conceived.*

*Dry again,
and a baby
cannot start
to grow.*

WHAT DOES THE MUCUS FEEL LIKE?

FERTILE: A wet feeling similar to the beginning of menstruation. Learn to sense the wetness of slippery mucus as you go about your daily activities.

FERTILE: Wet, sticky, pasty, smooth or creamy

Sometimes fertile mucus is creamy or milky, like hand lotion, mayonnaise, or thin flour-and-water paste.

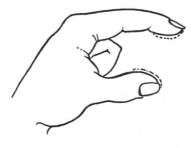

FERTILE: Wet, slippery, lubricative, sometimes stretchy

Sometimes fertile mucus is slippery, clear and stretchy, like raw egg-white. It may stretch into a thread or string between your fingers.

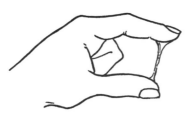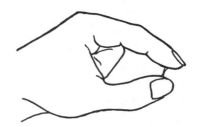

DRY

Rub your finger and thumb together to feel the "dry, no mucus" sensation.

You must feel dry from morning until evening to consider it a "dry day." Most dry days are infertile, but the first four dry days in a row after the mucus ends are fertile.

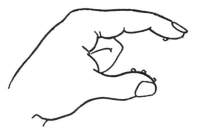

FERTILE

wet
creamy, pasty
milky
smooth, oily, greasy
like hand lotion
like mayonnaise
slippery
lubricative
egg white
stretches into a string
elastic, springy

Colors

white, cloudy, clear
yellowish
pink, brown, or red
  (blood-tinged)

Odor

sweet

Taste

sweet (contains glucose,
  to nourish the sperm)

DRY

dry, no mucus
dense
stiff or crumbly
forms jagged stiff peaks
  on fingers

Colors

white or yellowish

Odor

musty

Taste

salty

FINDING THE MUCUS

1. Be aware of your body as you go about your daily activities. Does your vaginal area feel wet or dry? When the fertile mucus is present, it may feel almost like the beginning of your menstrual flow.

2. Find the mucus by **wiping downward once** across the vaginal opening *before and after* each visit to the toilet. Observing the mucus takes about 10 seconds or less per bathroom visit.

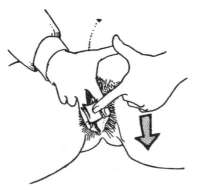

Wipe with your clean fingertip, or white, unscented toilet tissue.

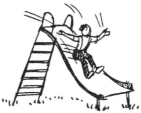

3. Does wiping feel dry, stiff, wet, smooth, slippery, lubricative?

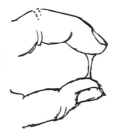

4. Touch mucus on the tissue or your fingers. Does the mucus look crumbly, creamy, milky, clear, stretchy, blood-tinged? Is there nothing to see?

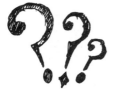

5. Are there any *changes* from your other observations today or yesterday? More, wetter, more lubricative or stretchier mucus indicates increasing fertility.

6. Just before bedtime, do a few *"Kegel exercises"* before your last observation of the day. Tighten and release your vaginal muscles a few times as if stopping and starting the flow of urine. Then bear down. Wipe and observe your mucus. Some women find the only fertile mucus of the day after doing the Kegels.

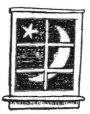

7. *Record your observations* on a chart before bedtime. Recording takes about 10-30 seconds.

(Please do not depend on memory. A woman is only following the ovulation method if she is checking often and charting every day.)

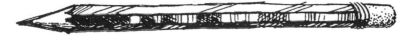

THE TYPICAL MUCUS PATTERN

Menstrual period. Considered fertile since the slippery blood can hide the beginning of slippery fertile mucus.

Dry days. When every observation is dry, all day long, you are infertile that evening. To avoid pregnancy, do not make love in the morning, because the mucus may have already begun, or might start later that day.

Fertile days. Wetness, lubrication, or any mucus or spotting *even once*, signal fertility. You will be fertile until the evening of the fourth dry day in a row afterwards.

Fourth dry day after the mucus ends. The evening of the fourth dry day in a row is infertile.

Dry days after ovulation. Infertile at any time of day or night until menstruation begins.

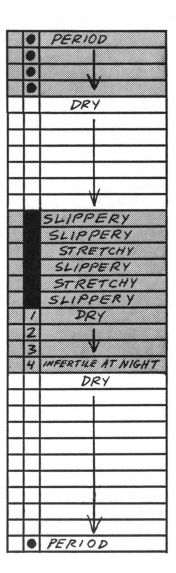

Tips on Finding the Mucus

Check before and after urination and especially after a bowel movement, which frequently brings down mucus.

When you dab yourself dry after urinating, look on the toilet tissue — you'll often see pieces of fertile mucus there.

After intercourse, doing the Kegel exercise will expel excess seminal fluid, making mucus observations easier.

Kegel exercises strengthen the muscles of the pelvic floor. Strengthened muscles increase a woman's enjoyment during intercourse, and can also help alleviate a problem with urinating involuntarily while running, laughing or sneezing.

Attention swimmers! Swimming may dry up external mucus for a few hours, but you will be fertile the whole time. You may check internally throughout the day, by placing a finger within the vagina. The changes are obvious: infertile (sticky or stiff), then wet, slippery and/or stretchy fertile mucus, and back to infertile stickiness. And be sure to do the Kegel exercise each evening (p. 25). If you wish, use temperature to confirm that your fertile phase is finished.

Check before bathing, showering, and swimming.

Also check after exercising and whenever you sense wetness or the sliding sensation of the mucus.

Charting

Just before bedtime, **record the most fertile appearing observation of the day.** For instance, if you were dry almost all day, but there was wet creamy mucus once, record *"wet creamy mucus."* If you had slippery or stretchy mucus just once, write down *"slippery, stretchy mucus."* Describe the mucus in your own words.

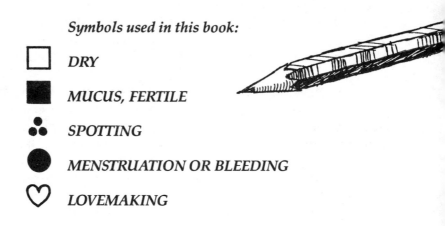

Symbols used in this book:

☐ *DRY*

■ *MUCUS, FERTILE*

∴ *SPOTTING*

● *MENSTRUATION OR BLEEDING*

♡ *LOVEMAKING*

About mucus descriptions

Some mucus descriptions, such as "sticky mucus" mean something different to every person. So don't worry about terminology. Just notice how you yourself change from dryness to wetness and lubrication, and back to dryness. Then you'll know when you're fertile and when you're not.

Using the charts in this book

Most charts in this book illustrate nearly all the days on which lovemaking would not result in pregnancy. Those charts explaining how to become pregnant show a few of the most likely days for getting pregnant. In reality, a couple may or may not make love on every day indicated in this book.

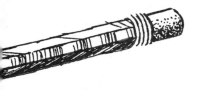

Where can I find charts to use?

There are blank charts at the back of this book. You may photocopy them, order more from the publisher, or design your own.

Invent a chart that suits you

Blind women sometimes use a string of differently shaped beads to keep track of the dry and mucus days. Women who cannot read may just draw a row of symbols instead of written descriptions. In cultures around the world where the people do not read or write, women successfully keep track of their mucus using beads of different colors.

If making observations is physically difficult

A woman could have her partner check her mucus if she does not have the use of her hands.

DRY DAYS BEFORE OVULATION

As your menstrual bleeding ends, there may be some spotting. If you observe dryness all day, you are infertile that evening.

After menstruation and spotting end, most women have some days which are dry all day long. The number of dry days varies from cycle to cycle, and from woman to woman. Some cycles do not have any dry days at all before ovulation.

On dry days, you may make love on **alternate evenings**. The day after intercourse, you will probably be wet and slippery from lovemaking. On the following day you will be able to make observations without any slippery fluids from intercourse.

	●	MENSTRUATION
	●	HEAVY BLEEDING
	●	MEDIUM BLEEDING
	●	MEDIUM BLEEDING
♡	∴	SPOTTING – DRY
		DRY
♡		DRY
		DRY
♡		DRY
		DRY
♡		DRY

Q. What is a dry day?

A. Dry all day long.

Q. When may you make love on dry days before ovulation, in order to avoid pregnancy?

A. Alternate evenings.

On dry days before ovulation avoid lovemaking in the morning. Your mucus may have already begun the night before. Or fertile mucus might appear later in the day, signaling fertility.

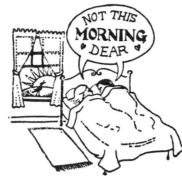

Morning sex and men

Some men are more in the mood for intercourse in the morning, when their sexual hormones are at the highest level. Instead of waiting until morning, a couple could make a point of scheduling lovemaking for the evening. Together, they may seek other ways to express their cooperation and satisfy a craving for affection in the early hours. (Some suggestions are listed in the *Practical Strategies* chapter). After the fertile phase, lovemaking at any time of the day or night will not cause a pregnancy.

Eliminating excess fluids

After intercourse, you may reduce the amount of seminal fluid by doing Kegel exercises (tightening and releasing the vaginal muscles as if starting and stopping the flow of urine). Without excess fluids from intercourse, mucus observations are clearer.

Consecutive evenings

After about three cycles, you'll be able to easily differentiate mucus, semen and arousal fluid from your cervical mucus. If seminal and vaginal fluids have dried up in the morning and you are totally dry for at least 10 hours, you may make love on consecutive nights.

FERTILE DAYS AND NIGHTS

If you happen to **see** spotting, wet creamy mucus, or stretchy pieces of mucus, you are fertile.

You might not see any mucus. If you merely **feel** slippery wetness, you are fertile.

You will be fertile until the evening of the fourth dry day in a row after the mucus, slippery wetness or spotting end.

To avoid pregnancy, avoid all genital-to-genital contact on any fertile day or night. This means refrain from sexual intercourse, as well as "early withdrawal."

INFERTILE DAYS AND NIGHTS

The evening of the fourth dry day in a row after slippery wetness or spotting end is infertile. Beginning then, you may make love at any time of day or night until menstruation begins, as long as the mucus remains dry.

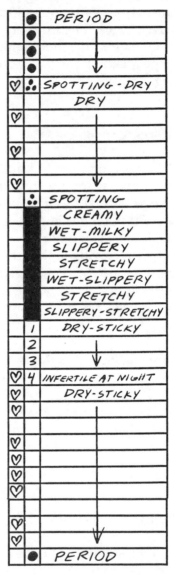

To avoid pregnancy on fertile days or nights, avoid getting a drop of the man's semen on the inside or even the outside of the vagina. The millions of sperm cells in that one drop can swim up the channels in the fertile mucus, and may cause a pregnancy.

Intercourse with barrier methods sometimes results in pregnancy during the fertile phase. If any sperm escape the spermicidal cream or foam, the mucus can keep them alive until ovulation.

Q. If you feel wet or slippery when wiping, but you do not see any mucus, are you fertile?   A. Yes.

Q. If you feel dry when wiping, but you see some mucus or spotting, are you fertile?   A. Yes.

Q. If you see or feel slippery wet mucus or spotting just once during the day, are you fertile?   A. Yes.

Q. Once the mucus ends, when will you be infertile again?
A. On the evening of the fourth dry day in a row.

The "Peak day" and ovulation

The last day of any mucus is sometimes called the "Peak day." Ovulation usually happens on the Peak day, or the day after. About 10-15% of the time, women ovulate two or rarely three days before or after the mucus ends.[2]

After ovulating, the egg lives and can be fertilized for 12-24 hours. But remember, every day of mucus is potentially fertile since the mucus will sustain sperm cells until the egg is ready.

BECOMING PREGNANT

Now that you know when you are the most fertile, you may plan a pregnancy when you wish.

If you would like to become pregnant, the days and nights of abundant wet, slippery or stretchy mucus are the times to make love.

The last mucus day and the day after are usually the most fertile of all. <u>Also</u> make love on the <u>second day after the mucus ends.</u>

The mucus will keep sperm cells alive for 3-5 days until ovulation, so you don't need to make love on every mucus day. In fact, it's highly recommended to *wait a day or so before making love again*, to allow 40-48 hours for your partner's sperm count to increase.

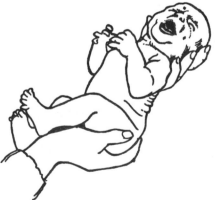

●	PERIOD	
●		
●		
●		
⁂	SPOTTING-DRY	
	DRY	
⁂	SPOTTING	
	CREAMY	
	WET-MILKY	
♡	SLIPPERY	
	STRETCHY	
♡	WET-SLIPPERY	
	STRETCHY	
♡	SLIPPERY-STRETCHY	
♡	1	DRY-STICKY
	2	
	3	
	4	
	PREGNANT	

Infrequent fertile phases

A woman might wait for months or years to see or feel fertile mucus. Once it is there, even for a few hours, the mucus signals her most fertile time.

Conception date and due date

Sometimes due dates are determined using outdated rhythm calculations: counting seven days from the last period, then back three months. Such guesswork assumes you ovulated on day 14. It is more accurate to base your calculations on the mucus. Even if a couple makes love on the early days of mucus, conception itself happens later on when the egg ovulates. Ovulation usually happens on the last mucus day or the day after. The baby's due date is 266 days after conception, plus or minus six days.

Confirming pregnancy naturally

If there is no menstruation 17 days after *obvious* fertile mucus ends, you are probably pregnant. A continuously high basal body temperature for 17 days after obvious mucus ends confirms pregnancy, unless you are ill and have a fever. (See the *Temperature* chapter.)

Throughout pregnancy, the temperature will remain high due to progesterone, the "hormone of pregnancy."

How long will it take?

A couple of normal fertility might make love during one to six or more fertile phases before becoming pregnant.

Q. To get pregnant, when should a couple make love?

A. Whenever there is wet, slippery or stretchy mucus, a woman is potentially fertile. The most fertile days of all are the last mucus day, *and* the first one or two days after the mucus ends.

Q. Should couples make love every day when there is mucus?

A. No, it is recommended to wait 40-48 hours in between to allow the man's sperm count to replenish.

Q. Can a woman get pregnant by making love on days of wet, creamy, pasty mucus, or when there is hardly any mucus?

A. Yes, women do get pregnant from lovemaking on days of sticky, creamy, pasty or scant mucus.

Q. What kind of mucus is most fertile?

A. Abundant, wet, stretchy, clear mucus is very fertile. However, even just a little wetness or mucus enables women to get pregnant.

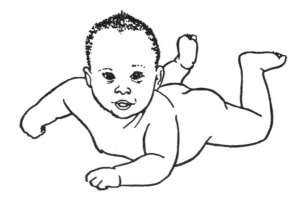

DELAYED OVULATION (Stress Cycles)

Unusual stress may cause you to ovulate later than usual. Your mucus will build up, taper off, and then a few days or weeks later, the mucus will begin again.

Sometimes the first mucus patch doesn't seem quite as slippery or obvious as usual. Keep watching for fertile mucus to begin.

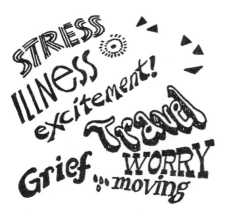

You will actually ovulate only once per cycle, as the final fertile mucus patch ends. Menstruation will begin 10-16 days after you ovulate.

If you are uncertain about your mucus, a temperature chart is handy for confirming that ovulation is over. *See the Temperature chapter.*

	●	PERIOD
	●	
	●	↓
♡	⁚	DRY
		GRIEF
♡		DRY
		↓
♡		TRAVEL
		STAYING UP ALL NIGHT
		SLICK
		SMOOTH
		↓
	⁚	SPOTTING
		DAMP
		↓
		CREAMY
		STRETCHY
		↓
	1	DRY
	2	
	3	↓
		STRETCHY
		↓
	1	DRY-STICKY
	2	
	3	↓
♡	4	INFERTILE AT NIGHT
♡		DRY STICKY
♡		
♡		
♡		
♡		
♡		
♡		↓
	●	PERIOD

*Some types of stress which often cause
delayed ovulation:*

travel	*a new job*
excitement	*losing or gaining weight rapidly*
worry	*more exercise than usual*
illness	*sudden change in diet*
moving	*going away to school*
family problems	*working on a big project*
grief	*having house guests*
	preparing for holiday celebrations

Natural fertility control continues to work

Your own body and its fertility signs react to stress in predictable ways. So there is no point in getting discouraged with the ovulation method because of early or delayed ovulation. The mucus will be honest with you. Be honest with yourself and your partner; talk the situation over and decide on a plan for avoiding pregnancy while your mucus signals are temporarily confusing.

The cause of delayed ovulation

Your hypothalamus gland, which masterminds the timing of ovulation, is very sensitive to emotions, light, diet, and other stresses. So stress can make the hypothalamus change your expected time of ovulation. You may be able to alter the effects of stress on your system through exercise, diet, relaxation exercises or affirmations. *See page 126.*

Q. Are you now experiencing any stressful events which might change the timing of your fertile phase? Can you anticipate some in the future?

1.

2.

3.

Q. If your mucus is confusing and ovulation is delayed, what do you and your partner plan to do?

1. One general rule for using natural methods is *"When in doubt, wait."*

2. Natural methods encourage you to find loving alternatives to intercourse. *For ideas, see the Practical Strategies chapter.*

3. Some couples do not continue using natural methods; instead they temporarily turn to barrier methods which usually, though not always, prevent pregnancy.

4. Others may "hope" or "assume" they aren't fertile, and make love. Naturally, pregnancy can result.

SHORT CYCLES

Fertile mucus can begin while you menstruate. The slippery menstrual blood can hide the presence of slippery mucus. So all days of menstruation are considered fertile.

Once your bleeding lightens, you will notice whether you are dry all day, or whether you have wet, slippery mucus.

Wet slippery days are **fertile**. To avoid pregnancy, avoid intercourse and genital-to-genital contact until the evening of the fourth dry day in a row after the mucus and bleeding end.

●	PERIOD	
●		
●		
●	↓	
∴	SPOTTING - WET	
∴	↓	
■	WET - SLIPPERY	
■	STRETCHY	
■	WET - SLIPPERY	
1	DRY	
2		
3		
♡ 4		
♡		
♡		
♡		
♡		
♡		
♡		
♡		
♡	↓	
●	PERIOD	

Any woman may have an occasional short cycle, especially if she is under unusual stress or nearing menopause. So even though you may have had 10 years of long cycles, the next cycle could be short. You can avoid surprises by observing your mucus regularly whenever you visit the bathroom.

SPOTTING OR BLEEDING

Spotting at the end of your menstrual period is infertile **if you are dry all day.**

Any non-menstrual spotting during other parts of your cycle indicates **possible fertility.** Spotting may be pink, brown or red.

Consider yourself fertile until the evening of the fourth dry day in a row after the spotting ends. If you did not actually have any wet, slippery fertile mucus yet, you may not have ovulated, so keep watching.

Unusual bleeding

●		PERIOD
●		↓
♡	:•	SPOTTING - DRY
	:•	SPOTTING - DRY
♡		DRY
♡		↓
	:•	SPOTTING
	••	↓
	1	DRY
	2	
	3	
♡	4	
		↓
	■	WET-MILKY
	■	CREAMY
	■	STRETCHY
		↓
	:•	SPOTTING
	1	DRY
	2	
	3	
♡	4	
♡		↓

"Unusual bleeding" outside of the regular menstrual period commonly happens to women who are breast-feeding, pre-menopausal, or coming off the Pill. In addition, ovarian cysts or other health problems cause irregular bleeding or spotting which is not like normal menstruation. Discuss any unusual bleeding with your health practitioner.

Cyclic bleeding and D.E.S.

If your mother took the drug D.E.S. (diethylstilbestrol) while she was pregnant with you, you may have cyclic recurrent bleeding or spotting. Your mucus chart can document cyclic, regularly occurring "unusual bleeding," allowing you to avoid unnecessary medications or treatment.

ANOVULATORY CYCLES

Once in a while, you may not even ovulate. If no egg is released, the cycle is infertile.

Mucus will be watery, "in-between," and not really as slippery and obvious as usual.

Patience is recommended. Whenever you are unsure about your mucus, it's wise to assume you are fertile.

Long-distance runners or ballet dancers often experience anovulatory cycles with light periods. Vegetarians or others who restrict their intake of fats and protein are also prone to anovulatory cycles. And anorexic or bulimic women often experience anovulation. Depending on her circumstances, a woman may eat more unprocessed, unsaturated vegetable oils and protein, or gradually cut down on exercise until ovuluation resumes.

●		PERIOD
●		
●		
●		
●		
♡	∴	SPOTTING- DRY
		DRY
♡		
		DAMP
		WATERY
	1	DRY
		SLICK
	1	DRY
	2	
		DAMP
		WATERY
		MILKY
	1	DRY
		PASTY
		SLIPPERY
		WET
	1	DRY
		WET
	1	DRY

If ovulation does not occur, the temperature will stay relatively low throughout the usual cycle. Menstruation may be heavy, light, or might not even happen, depending on the cause of anovulation.

During pregnancy, a woman will not ovulate. She will feel dry, stiff, sticky mucus and her temperature will be high.

INFERTILE PATTERN
OF CONSTANT UNCHANGING MUCUS

You may observe a small amount of pasty, sticky, *dry* mucus discharge which is exactly the same day after day.

Please chart carefully for three complete cycles, and ask an ovulation method teacher what to do if you have constant discharges. Teachers are listed near the end of the book.

CONSTANTLY CHANGING MUCUS

Gummy mucus, or lots of mucus that changes from day to day can result from a cervix damaged by surgery, disease, or exposure to the drug diethylstilbestrol (D.E.S.) while you were in your mother's womb.

When your mucus changes constantly, a temperature chart can be especially helpful. Also contact an ovulation method teacher for assistance. She may be able to help you distinguish fertile mucus from your other discharges.

If the discharge is smelly and irritating, you probably have a vaginal infection (see the *Vaginal Infections* chapter for remedies). Odorless, non-irritating discharges might signal a medical problem. If there is no medical problem the discharge itself does not require medical treatment. With practice, many women can tell the difference between slippery fertile mucus and a day-to-day discharge.

Unless you have severe cervical problems such as cancer, avoid undergoing a *cone biopsy*. Also called *conization*, the procedure will destroy cervical crypts. Fewer crypts means less mucus, lowered fertility, and more difficulty identifying your fertile phase.

It's normal for cycles to vary.

Amounts of mucus normally vary from cycle to cycle. Even a very tiny amount of fertile mucus can help conception occur.

You may ovulate early in one cycle, late in the next, etc. Your mucus will tell when you are fertile.

SLIPPERY DISCHARGE BEFORE MENSTRUATION

In some cycles you may notice a wet, slippery, stretchy or clear discharge a few days before menstruation. If you already had an *obvious* fertile phase, the discharge is infertile.

But think back...were you under stress earlier in your cycle? If you were, fertile appearing mucus could have begun earlier, stopped, and now may be starting again.

A temperature chart will confirm whether or not the discharge is fertile. See the *Temperature* chapter.

	●	PERIOD
	●	
	●	
	●	
♡	∴	SPOTTING – DRY
		DRY
♡		
		STRETCHY
	1	CREAMY
	2	STIFF, CREAMY
	3	STIFF
♡	4	
♡		
♡		
♡		
♡		
♡		CREAMY
♡		
♡		CREAMY STRETCHY
♡		CLEAR
	●	PERIOD

CYCLE LENGTHS AND MENSTRUATION

Menstruation almost always begins 10-16 days (about two weeks) after the mucus ends. It is the number of days before ovulation which varies, resulting in cycles of different lengths.

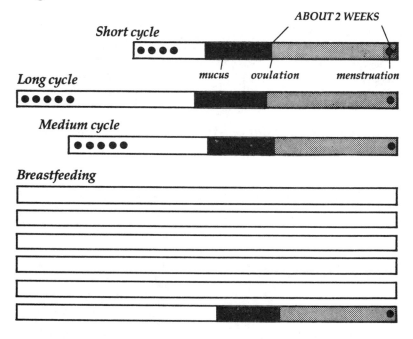

Long, short, and irregular cycles are all perfectly normal. If you wish, you may experiment with regulating your cycle length using light (p. 84) in order to have 29-31 day cycles, shorter but heavier menstruation, and a more distinct mucus pattern.

During pre-menopause, or when fertility resumes after breastfeeding or stopping contraceptive pills, the post-ovulatory days may vary in number for a few cycles.

Mucus usually lasts about 3-9 days (average 6 days). Menstrual bleeding is generally 3-7 days (average 5 days). Mucus for more than 10 days may reflect a health problem or allergy. Check with a teacher who's experienced in advanced case management *(pp. 136-138)*.

Your Temperature Signal

A woman's temperature in the morning, right after she awakens, is low between menstruation and ovulation. Around the time of ovulation, the temperature rises and remains high for about two weeks until the next menstrual period. The hormone estrogen helps cause the low temperatures before ovulation. Higher temperatures reflect the higher levels of progesterone hormone secreted after ovulation.

You may use your temperature chart to identify infertile days after ovulation.

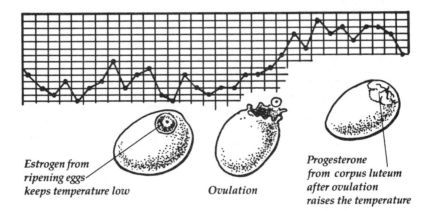

Estrogen from ripening eggs keeps temperature low

Ovulation

Progesterone from corpus luteum after ovulation raises the temperature

There is no such thing as a "typical" temperature chart

Even if your temperature chart differs wildly from other charts you have seen, it is still completely normal. After studying over 20,000 temperature charts, Dr. Rudolph Vollman concluded that every woman's graph is unique to her.[1] And there is no particular point on the graph which indicates the day of ovulation.

46

Mucus only, or mucus plus temperature?

You can use mucus alone for effective fertility control if you wish. Many women find this the simplest method.

If you prefer, you may add temperature to your mucus observations. Using both the mucus and temperature signals is known as the *"sympto-thermal method."*

When to use temperature

Confidence building. The temperature chart may help you feel more confident as you learn your mucus pattern. Your temperature can also help you decide if a slippery discharge just before menstruation is fertile or not.

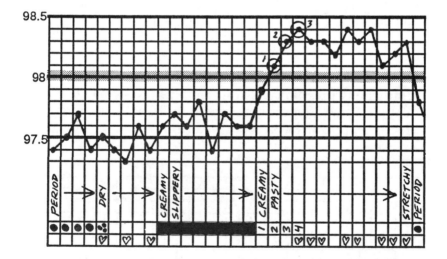

After the Pill. After a woman has stopped taking oral contraceptives, she may have weeks on end of wet, confusing mucus. Temperature can be the clearest sign that ovulation is over and that the infertile phase has begun.

Becoming pregnant. If your temperature stays low until a day or two after your last mucus, you may be ovulating *after* the mucus ends. Be sure to have intercourse on the one or two days after the mucus ends, since there is not as much mucus available to assist in sperm survival.

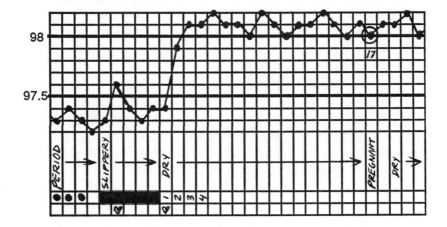

Confirming pregnancy. If your temperature stays high for 17 days in a row after obvious mucus ends, and you do not menstruate, pregnancy is confirmed (unless you are ill and have a fever).

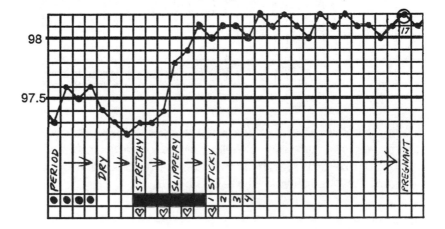

Delayed ovulation due to stress. Your temperature chart will indicate, by remaining low, that you have not yet ovulated. The temperature will also show when ovulation is over and you are no longer fertile (as will your mucus if you observe it carefully).

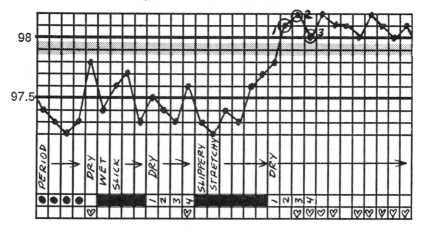

Corpus luteum problems. The hormone progesterone triggers high temperatures after ovulation. Progesterone is secreted by the *corpus luteum,* which was formerly the follicle surrounding the ripening egg. If your corpus luteum is not making enough progesterone to support a pregnancy, the temperature will drop and menstruation will begin nine or less days after the mucus ends.

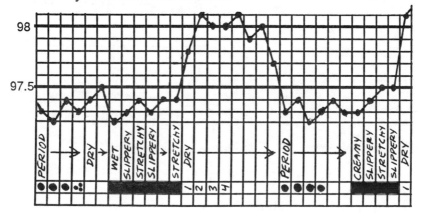

How to take your temperature

1. **As soon as you wake up each day,** take your temperature, before eating, drinking, smoking or brushing teeth. If possible, take the temperature at the same time daily.

2. **If using a mercury thermometer,** orally, put the thermometer under your tongue for three minutes. Do not talk until finished. If you need utmost accuracy, take the temperature rectally or vaginally for three minutes.

   Using a digital thermometer, orally or vaginally, takes only a minute or two, and saves wear and tear on your wrist from shaking down mercury. In addition, the digitals do not break as easily as glass thermometers.

3. **Record the temperature on your chart.** Note if you took the reading at a different time than usual. Also be sure to note if you have a fever, or if your sleep was disturbed.

   Taking your temperature at an unusual time, going to bed late, drinking alcohol, eating late, illness, exercise or using an electric blanket can alter your temperature readings. At these times, and when you are running a fever, *your temperature may not accurately reflect your fertility.*

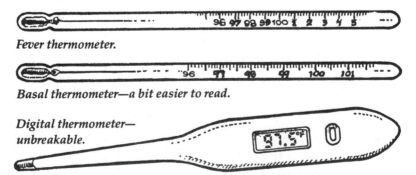

Fever thermometer.

Basal thermometer—a bit easier to read.

Digital thermometer— unbreakable.

   Excellent digital thermometers (with memory) can be ordered from **Barbara Feldman,** *The Fertility Awareness Center, P.O. Box 2606, New York, NY, USA 10009, $11 each.*

Interpreting your temperature chart

Here are instructions for one of the ways of interpreting the temperature chart.

1. Find the six low temperatures in a row just before the temperature starts to rise.

2. Draw a line one-tenth of a degree above the highest of the six low temperatures.

3. On the *evening* of the third temperature in a row *above that line,* you are probably infertile, unless your mucus shows fertility.

4. Of course you may wait another day if you wish to be even more careful.

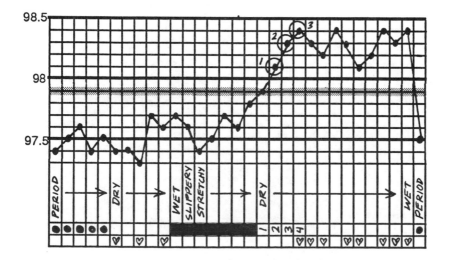

Your own basal body temperature may be far higher or lower than the temperatures depicted in this book.

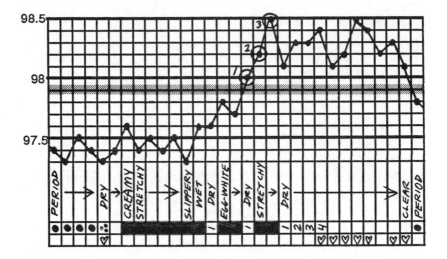

In this chart, temperature indicated infertility while the mucus still signaled fertility. Follow the mucus signal. *(Talk to a trained fertility awareness teacher about this type of chart, especially if you have mucus for more than 10 days. See p. 136.)*

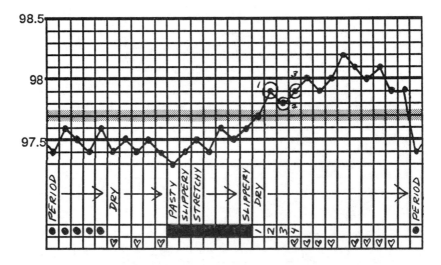

If it's not obvious which is the last day of low temperature, use the "Vollman method." Directions begin on the next few pages.

Using temperature alone

In order to use temperature alone, avoid intercourse before ovulation, and make love only after the temperature chart shows that ovulation and the fertile phase are over.

Using temperature alone is most useful after cervical surgery or damage, when you have a vaginal infection, or if you are temporarily confused about your mucus.

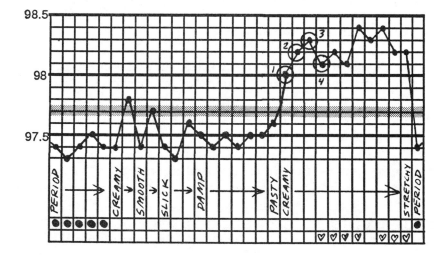

The mean-intercept method

This method was devised by Dr. Rudolf F. Vollman. It is usually considered one of the most accurate ways of using the temperature chart.

1. When your menstrual period begins, find the average of all the temperatures for the cycle which just ended. For example, if there were 32 days in your cycle, you would add all 32 temperatures together. Then you would divide the total by 32.

   (Obviously, you must have temperatures for one entire cycle — menstrual period to menstrual period — in order for the Vollman method to work.)

2. On the chart for your current cycle, draw a continuous line at that average temperature from your last cycle.

3. Find a new average for every cycle. Don't use an average from a few months or years ago.

4. On the *evening* of the third temperature in a row *above the line*, your infertility has begun.

5. However, if your *mucus* is slippery or you are in the midst of abstaining for four dry days, continue to follow the mucus guidelines no matter what your temperature says.

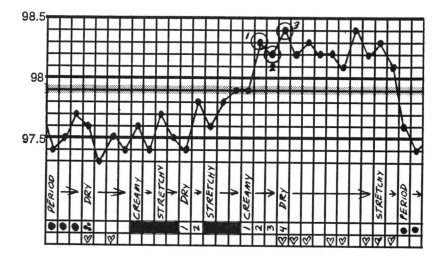

On the evening of the third temperature *above* the line, infertility begins, unless your mucus signals fertility.

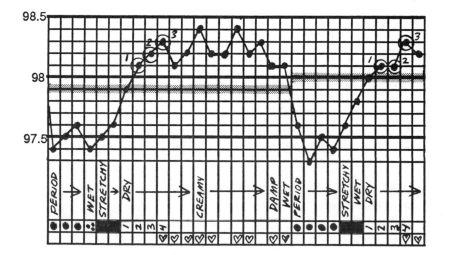

Find a new average for each cycle.

Energy, Moods, and Fertility Changes

By charting your moods, thoughts, emotions, and energy level along with your mucus observations, you may discover they are closely linked to your fertility changes. Although some women do not notice cyclic mood and energy variations, women who can predict such changes may plan work, activities, and family communication more effectively. Knowing when to expect physical and emotional changes also helps in the treatment of PMS (premenstrual syndrome).

As estrogen rises and ovulation approaches, many women report the following experiences:

- Increased sexual feelings, heightened desire, more feelings of affection. These feelings are important signals that fertility is at hand. It's no coincidence that the word *"estrogen,"* the fertility hormone, stems from Latin roots which mean *"creating mad desire."*

- High energy, easy concentration, much work accomplished. Less interest in sleeping and eating. Optimism, enthusiasm, clear, quick thinking.

- Clear soft radiant skin visible to others as well as the woman herself. Feelings of wetness, fullness and openness in the vaginal region, noticed by the woman and/or her partner.

- Easy magnetism, conversation, and increased confidence and sociability.

- Sexual dreams or dreams about babies. An interior voice calling or praying for a baby when making love immediately before or during the fertile phase.

- Elation and a definite sense of fertility which women themselves feel signifies ovulation.

After ovulation

As the fertile phase ends, women may report suddenly feeling depressed or let-down. In fact, some identify the beginning of their post-Peak phase with this emotional shift, in addition to the sudden absence of mucus. Sometimes sexual desire wanes, although many women have more desire during menstruation. Facial and body hair often grows faster and thicker.[1]

Record emotional and physical changes on your fertility chart. In your cycles, do the same moods or symptoms happen a particular number of days after the mucus ends?

Premenstrual syndrome

Many women are quite uncomfortable, emotionally and/or physically, before menstruation. After menstruation, they feel fine. These women have premenstrual syndrome, a physical condition which can be treated. Some of the common PMS symptoms are...

---

nervousness
irritability
angry outbursts
anxiety
mood swings
feeling out of control

    depression
    forgetfulness
    crying
    confusion
    feeling crazy

        weight gain
        swelling, water retention
        breast tenderness
        abdominal bloating

headaches
craving for sweets
   (especially chocolate)
increased appetite
fatigue
pounding heart
dizziness or fainting

        lack of coordination
        incoherent
        uninterested in sex
        more interested in sex
        acne
        lethargy
        constipation

Typical factors which precipitate PMS are hormonal, such as starting the Pill, quitting contraceptive Pills, giving birth, or tubal ligation (getting the "tubes tied"). Or, PMS may stem from stress, diet, or lack of exercise.

Self-help suggestions for alleviating PMS include

- Exercise at least 10 minutes a day.

- Cut down on sugar, salt, caffeine, and alcohol. Eat more fresh fruits, vegetables, and unrefined whole foods. Substitute flavorful uncaffeinated herbal teas for coffee.

- Do relaxation exercises, stretching, yoga, meditation, etc. daily.

- Schedule less stressful activities for low energy days. Plan activities requiring extra power during your fertile phase.

- Eat more foods high in Vitamin B_6, magnesium, and calcium. Examples include:
  B_6—rice bran, soybeans and other beans, fish, leafy greens, bananas, avocado, whole wheat or rye flour, raisins, cantaloupe, sunflower seeds (unroasted).[2]
  Calcium—milk products, leafy greens, sesame seed meal, broccoli, okra, tofu, soybeans, rutabaga.[3]
  Magnesium—beans, beet greens and other dark green leafy vegetables, buckwheat, whole wheat flour, cashews, almonds.[4]

- Involve those you live with. Tell them what you are trying to change and ask for their cooperation. For example, they could support your dietary changes, or help free some of your time so you can exercise.

- Vitamin supplements, progesterone therapy or other approaches may be recommended by your health practitioner. Record symptoms on your mucus/temperature chart, before, during and after treatment.

PMS is a reality for a large percentage of women

Not all women experience PMS, but those who do deserve support and should know PMS responds to treatment and self-help. By learning how to control the causes of PMS, we can "counteract the myth that all women should, by nature, be expected to go through regular periods of unpredictability and diminished competence."*

Managing moods

As you learn your own mood pattern, you may have the opportunity to plan important meetings, projects, or social occasions for your fertile phase, and to schedule less stressful activities for low energy days. One reader planned parties while she was fertile optimistic and very energetic. Two weeks later, the party date arrived to find her lethargic and grumpy, and just prior to menstruation. After a few cycles, she discovered the pattern, and now plans parties to coincide with her fertile, sociable phases.

Another started sudden arguments. The fighting subsided after about two days, for no apparent reason. Then she noticed that her anger always flared on the tenth or eleventh day after the mucus ended. She decided to pay more attention to troubling situations instead of just hoping they would go away. Then she could talk about the problems ahead of time, when she felt strongest, instead of exploding later on when she felt out of control.

Challenge your own negativity

The sheer strength of a negative mood can be channeled in a new, positive direction. One woman told the author, "Right before my period is the time I accomplish the most, nowadays. I simply got tired of my negative moods, and decided to change them into the most productive energy of my cycle."

*From "PMS: Premenstrual Syndrome" brochure, (Network Publications, a division of ETR Associates), Santa Cruz, CA

Practical Strategies

Apart from sterilization, avoiding intercourse while a woman is fertile is the surest way to avoid pregnancy. How can a couple generate the cooperation and love which will enhance their relationship during the fertile time while they postpone intercourse?

Deepening intimacy without intercourse

Here is a pleasant activity to share every day. Simply sit or lie quietly together for five minutes while looking into each others' eyes. Do not talk — just feel warm and close. Recall previous times you have felt intimate, or imagine how you would like to feel with your partner. Afterwards, share affection and take turns talking about how you felt.[1]

A one-minute-long hug every day also fosters intimacy.

Inviting cooperative communication

Try experimenting with conversation. First, both partners discuss abstinence or fertility for five minutes, phrasing everything in the form of a *question*. For the next five minutes, begin every statement with the word *"you."* For another five minutes, each statement begins with *"I,"* and at last, begin every sentence with *"we."* This exercise will help you discover which approaches antagonize and which ones invite cooperation and partnership.[2]

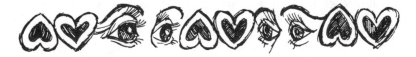

When a woman has been used to taking charge of fertility and contraception, sharing that control can be a new and challenging experience for both partners. Sometimes simply stating the facts, *"I am fertile today, I have fertile mucus today"* can invite a partner's cooperative response.

Men's participation

Most men are intrigued to discover the facts about their partner's fertility, and to know that they have an important role in cooperating and living harmoniously with it. A man's patience, love, and respect are priceless contributions to the couple's successful use of natural family planning.

He may also participate by checking the mucus (or having the woman show it to him), writing down the description, shaking down the thermometer, or coloring in the chart. Keeping the chart out in the open or in a special place encourages both partners to know which part of the cycle the woman — and thus the couple — is experiencing. The more informed both partners are, the easier it will be to share the decision to prevent or to try for pregnancy.

Postponing intercourse can foster intimacy and love

During the fertile period, each partner has the opportunity to reassure the other of their interest and regard, independent of their availability for intercourse. As a result, both partners feel prized for their sexuality as well as their other attributes.

Abstinence reminds partners how dearly they wish to be lovers. Avoiding intercourse can even restore romance in a relationship where sex is taken for granted. After trying it for awhile, many people are astounded by the communication and closeness that is generated.

Alternatives to intercourse

What are some of the loving activities you share through-out the day with your partner?

Try listing them, along with other romantic, physical, and non-physical ways which couples might use to sustain feel-ings of emotional closeness. Your list can include activities you yourself might not do, but which you have heard of or read about.

Some ways to share love and sexuality without intercourse

candle-light dinner
watch a movie
play music or sing together
look into each other's eyes
physical exercise
meditate or pray together
leave love notes for each other
buy or make gifts
read to each other
talk about feelings
   of love or desire

bathe together
massage each other
fantasize
dance
kiss, caress, etc.
  (Be creative. There are lots of ways to keep your sex life alive without inter-course.)

Write your own suggestions here:

1.

2.

3.

4.

5.

Talk about your feelings
on abstinence during the fertile phase.

Each partner may list his or her thoughts and feelings. Afterwards, exchange and share lists.

Positive aspects.	*Negative aspects.*
1.	1.
2.	2.
3.	3.
4.	4.
5.	5.
more...	**more...**

Role playing.

Either in a group, or at home, try role-playing. The woman pretends she is the man and the man pretends he is the woman while discussing abstinence. What is fertility awareness like from your partner's perspective?

One ovulation method class discussed how they felt about abstinence during the fertile time.[3] Here are their responses, word for word:

Negative

emotional frustration
requires planning, spontaneity gone or limited
no sex on special occasions if fertile
"sex on a schedule"
increased desire for sex at ovulation
frustrating
may bring about conflicts in relationship
not culturally acceptable
difficult for short term relationship
frightening responsibility
social pressure to have sex all the time
can require self-control you don't have
frustrating if fertility goes on for a long time
difficult to explain to partner
brings up unexpressed anger
afraid my partner is trying to avoid me
increases tension if partner doesn't want to cooperate

Positive

takes less energy
relief from contraceptives
good discipline
you get real horny and when you have sex it's special
don't take sex for granted
become more creative
increased communication between partners
helps to find a responsible mate
enjoy involvement of partner
increases self-esteem for woman who understands her body
partner learns more about your body and moods
    and can predict them better
strengthening for a relationship
experimenting with other ways of showing affection
communicating about our bodies
sharing responsibility
peace of mind during infertile periods
no encumbrances to sex
explore sexual alternatives to intercourse
not cancer producing
feels good spiritually and mentally
can get closer in touch with inner self
helps develop relationship with mate on other levels
explore new ways of making love
makes it a two person birth control method
don't have to support the contraceptive industry
safe, healthy
get a good night's sleep
approved by my religion
sparks creativity
feel cared for
increases desire
increases dream power
sure-fire birth control method
not changing anything in body
clarifies sexual feelings
natural and inexpensive
no side effects
anticipation sometimes better than the act itself

Celebrations

Every woman or couple who is using the natural methods will be likely at some time to have an overwhelming desire for intercourse even though it is during the fertile time. Being aware of these potential situations can help you plan ahead.[4] What will you and your partner do...

on a birthday
for Valentine's Day
during Christmas, New Year's Eve, or other holiday
after a fight or argument
before or after a trip or separation
whenever together, if you are rarely together
after seeing a romantic movie
on your wedding anniversary
while on vacation together
when undecided about pregnancy

Ways we could celebrate without intercourse...

1.

2.

3.

4.

5.

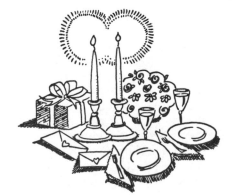

Challenges

During major life changes and transitions, a death in the family, or other times of loss, grief or uncertainty, a woman or couple may feel ambivalent about avoiding pregnancy, even though they had previously decided not to become pregnant. Together, discuss with your partner what you both might do...

during an emotional crisis
during a time of great stress
after a death of a parent or other family member
after a sibling has become pregnant or given birth
after deciding to have another child "in the future"

when changing jobs or careers
when just starting a new relationship
when contemplating ending an old relationship
when others pressure you to have children

while lonely or pleading for attention or help
when guessing about unclear fertility signs
while denying that pregnancy can happen to you
when needing to prove one's fertility
while trying to please your partner

What we might do during challenging times...

1.

2.

3.

4.

5.

Plans

What will you and your partner do to avoid pregnancy while you are fertile or unsure of your fertility?

Couples who wish to continue using natural methods are often motivated to find loving alternatives to intercourse until they are sure they are infertile.

Some couples decide to use a contraceptive barrier during the fertile period, instead of "taking a chance." Whenever couples use barriers, they are depending on the barrier alone to prevent pregnancy, and are not using the ovulation method nor the sympto-thermal method.

In addition, semen may escape the barrier and the spermicide into the protective mucus. Pregnancy can naturally result.

Strategies while fertile or unsure of the woman's fertility...

Least likelihood of pregnancy: Create and share romantic activities, and postpone intercourse.

Some chance of pregnancy: Contraceptive barriers and spermicides usually, but not always, prevent pregnancy.

High probability of pregnancy: "Hoping" the woman is not fertile and making love without barriers. Doing so may naturally result in pregnancy.

Our plans:

More practical strategies

Food affects your moods. Many people notice that their sex drive is higher after consuming alcohol or other foods. Avoiding these items may decrease the urgency to have intercourse, making it easier to refrain while fertile.

Reading. On a quiet note, an informative and inspiring book on abstinence and natural family planning is Mary Shivanandan's *Challenge to Love*, (KM Associates).

Form a support group. You may form a support group with the clients of a local teacher or teaching center, or with other friends who learn about the fertility signals from you.

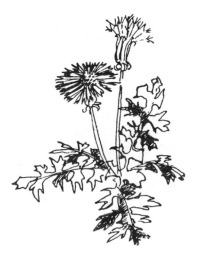

Arousal Fluid

Arousal fluid is the slippery liquid that your vagina secretes when you are sexually aroused or "turned on." You may feel wet arousal fluid when you have sexual thoughts or dreams, are touched in a way that makes you feel sexual, or while you are making love.

Intercourse will be painful without enough slippery arousal fluid, but you may buy lubricants to use if you don't seem to have enough of your own. (Use only water soluble lubricants; olive oil is even better. Never use petroleum jelly; it is petroleum based and harmful to your vaginal membranes.)

Affectionately increasing lubrication

Natural lubrication may increase when you and your partner kiss and caress lovingly and sexually for 20-60 minutes without intercourse. Sharing affection this way is especially important while breastfeeding and after menopause, when many women are naturally drier. Also keep olive oil or lubricant handy and ask your partner to use it automatically.

Non-sexual touching

You may also try taking turns touching each other in affectionate but non-sexual ways, avoiding breasts and genitals. Take 20 minutes to touch for your own pleasure, then devote 20 minutes to your partner's enjoyment. If partners haven't felt very aroused with each other in the past, gentle affectionate touching can be a way to begin feeling comfortable together. As you allow your sexual feelings to develop unhurriedly, natural lubrication will often flow more easily.

Distinguishing arousal fluid from cervical mucus

Sometime when you are aroused, wipe across the vulva as you do when observing your mucus. You'll feel very lubricative as you wipe; slippery cervical mucus can feel exactly the same way.

Try to pick up some of the slippery fluid. It is much more *watery* than cervical mucus, and has *less substance*. If you stretch it between your fingers, the arousal fluid will usually be very thin and will break apart. It rarely stretches more than two times, and usually disappears from the vagina within a few hours. And arousal fluid will easily dissolve in water.

Cervical mucus, by comparison, *has more substance*. Even a tiny piece can be picked up, stretched repeatedly, and held stretched out for many seconds. Visible cervical mucus is more like a "thing," — almost like a shred of gelatin dessert or the thick part of an egg white. Fertile mucus is also more oily than arousal fluid, and clumps up under water.

Sometimes fertile mucus will make you feel slippery even though there is no mucus to be seen. If wiping feels slippery, consider yourself fertile.

Within two or three cycles, you will be able to easily distinguish cervical mucus from arousal fluid.

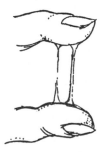

**When in doubt,
assume you are fertile.**

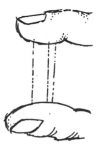

Cervical mucus   **Arousal fluid**

Breastfeeding

A mother will be naturally
infertile for some time after
giving birth, while her baby
eats and drinks nothing except
the mother's own milk. When the
baby sucks on the breast, the woman's
prolactin hormone is released. Prolactin
stimulates milk production and generally inhibits ovulation.

Ovulation resumes — sometimes very quickly — when the
baby sucks less often, sleeps through the night, or demands
less breast milk. **Some women ovulate even while the baby
is still totally breastfeeding.** Heavier and better nourished
women generally resume ovulating sooner than women
who are thinner.

72

Breastfeeding and the fertility signals

Fertility awareness is especially valuable for nursing mothers because regular cycles are not necessary. The mucus will signal whether or not a breastfeeding woman is fertile each day.

Fertility may be delayed for months or years while breastfeeding. As fertility returns, wet, slippery mucus or spotting will signal possible fertility. The mucus may start and stop a few times before a woman finally ovulates.

If she wishes, a woman may take her temperature each morning when the mucus patches begin. Temperature can signal that ovulation actually did take place at the end of one of the mucus build-ups. After ovulation, menstruation will begin within about two weeks.

Sometimes menstruation begins less than two weeks after ovulation during the first few cycles of renewed fertility. After a while, cycles return to their normal length.

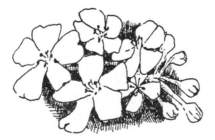

When does fertility return without breastfeeding?

A woman will usually be fertile within four to six weeks after a miscarriage, abortion, or live-birth if she does not breastfeed.

WHAT TO DO

Begin charting as soon as the baby is born

Once your bleeding (lochia) subsides after birth, take two weeks to chart your breastfeeding pattern carefully. Follow the instructions on pages 20-36 for observing and using the mucus. Refrain from intercourse during these two weeks so that the slippery fluids from lovemaking will not confuse your observations.

You will identify your *"infertile breastfeeding pattern."* This is the pattern which, for two weeks in a row, remains *exactly the same* in texture, moisture, color, amount and sensation at the vulva (vaginal opening). Any CHANGE from this pattern, for example, more mucus, more wetness or lubrication, stretchiness, clarity, spotting or bleeding, is considered FERTILE. After fertile signs end, wait until the evening of the fourth day in a row of your infertile pattern. Then continue to make love on alternate evenings. Do not make love in the morning, because you don't know if fertile signs will begin again later that day.

The usual breastfeeding patterns

DRY EVERY DAY. Anything else, such as creamy, sticky mucus, stretchiness, clarity, dampness, lubrication, spotting or bleeding, signals possible fertility. Wait until the evening of the fourth dry day in a row, then resume lovemaking on alternate evenings.

PASTY, DRY, STICKY MUCUS EVERY DAY. Any *change*— more dampness, lubrication, clarity, stretchiness, spotting or bleeding, signals potential fertility. On the evening of the fourth day in a row of the usual pasty mucus, lovemaking can resume on alternate evenings.

CONTINUOUS WET MILKY DISCHARGE. It is not slippery, not stretchy, has no substance, and dries to nothing. Any change from this signals fertility.

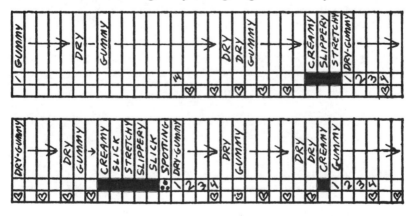

MOSTLY DRY DAYS, with a few days of discharge. The days of discharge are considered fertile. Wait until the evening of the fourth dry day in a row to resume intercourse on alternate dry evenings.

UNCHANGING DISCHARGE ON MOST DAYS, with a few dry days here and there. Whenever the discharge is present it is *exactly the same.* If no bleeding starts within two weeks of the unchanging discharge, it didn't signal fertility. So the dry days and the days of unvarying discharge are infertile in the evening. Any *change* signals fertility.

What is happening?

Sucking on the breast stimulates the hormone prolactin which serves to keep estrogen levels low. An unchanging infertile pattern results. When there is less suckling, estrogen levels increase, and the mucus pattern naturally changes to something else—increasing in quantity, lubrication, stretchiness, clarity, spotting or bleeding. The mucus changes signal greater fertility.

During breastfeeding, estrogen levels may rise and fall many times before triggering ovulation. Each time, slippery mucus will let you know you are potentially fertile. The mucus which signals ovulation may be less abundant or less stretchy than during your usual cycles, but it will still have the obviously lubricative feeling of "the real thing."

Once menstruation begins

When you finally ovulate, true menstruation will start about two weeks later. Then take two weeks to watch for your new infertile pattern, using directions on pages 20-33. Remember that although a discharge may have been considered infertile during breastfeeding, during your regular cycles a similar discharge will signal *fertility*.

Hints

Please call or write to a teacher (pages 136-138) if you are confused, have a continuous wet slippery discharge, or mucus which varies from day to day. Pay special attention to the feeling of dryness, wetness or lubrication at your vulva (as a blind woman would) to more surely sense changes or similarities from day to day.

Part of the breastfeeding response is the production of arousal fluid *(see pp. 70-71)*. You'll notice continual wetness or dampness. Be sure to check mucus about a half-hour before anticipated nursing, and if possible a few hours later. You'll probably have the "continuous wet milky discharge" pattern *(page 75)*.

At about three months a *new* infertile breastfeeding pattern may develop. Identify it by watching for two weeks just as you did at the start of breastfeeding.

Giving birth can irritate or damage the cervix, and constant discharges are the result. Have your doctor check your cervix.

Prolonging natural infertility

At six or nine months, your baby may have a growth spurt and seem to nurse less, or need more milk than you can supply. If you can, take a day or two to rest, drink extra liquids (non-caffeinated) and nurse frequently whenever the baby wishes, especially at night. Frequent breastfeeding usually helps increase the milk supply, and natural infertility often continues. Ask your family for their cooperation which will enable you to take the needed rest.

SIGNS OF RETURNING FERTILITY

increased sexual desire	*elastic/stretchy mucus*
higher energy levels	*clear mucus*
more mucus	*spotting or bleeding*
wetter, more slippery mucus	

FERTILITY MAY BE ON ITS WAY WHEN...

the baby sleeps through the night
there is a longer time between feedings
bottle feeding begins
you work outside the home
the baby sucks on a pacifier (instead of your breast)
the baby is teething
you or the baby are traveling, irritable, ill, or under stress

---

You DO NOT necessarily need to stop nursing if you want to conceive again. That's a myth! Just eliminate one nursing per day, watch for mucus, and see if you are getting fertile. Gradually taper off nursing just enough to become fertile. Mucus may start and stop many times during the weeks before you finally ovulate. Regular, frequent mucus observations, plus cooperation with your partner are invaluable in controlling the timing of another pregnancy - whether you want to conceive now, or not.

Sexual desire suddenly increases

Many women report that their sex drive increases dramatically as their estrogen level rises before ovulation. Sexual desire while fertile could be thought of as nature's way of helping couples conceive another baby at the first available opportunity.

In order to use natural methods to avoid another pregnancy, both partners may list or discuss some romantic and creative alternatives to intercourse, so that they will be prepared when the fertile phase begins.

Some couples temporarily stop using natural methods, and turn to barrier methods if the woman is unsure of her fertility while breastfeeding. They understand that pregnancies occasionally occur while couples use contraceptive barriers during the fertile time, since the mucus can aid sperm survival. Other couples who feel suddenly more sexual than they have in months, may "hope" they are not fertile, and make love without barriers. Naturally, pregnancy often results. **What will you do?**

Weaning

Once the baby is weaned, your mucus pattern will return to normal within a few weeks. If your breastfeeding pattern was of continuous unchanging mucus, you may have a new pattern after breastfeeding ends. Any wet, smooth, slippery and/or stretchy mucus, or spotting, signals possible fertility.

Avoid oral contraceptives

Taking the regular or the progesterone-only Pill while nursing is totally inadvisable. Your baby should not be ingesting adult female hormones from the Pill which will be secreted into your breast milk. Moreover, why take a fertility suppressing drug every day when breastfeeding stimulates nature's own infertility hormone — prolactin — and the mucus signal will predict when your fertility is returning?

Breastfeeding and sex

Breastfeeding can totally change sexual relationships, giving couples an opportunity to rediscover each other and create new approaches to sex. The woman may have much less energy and desire, and extreme vaginal dryness will make intercourse painful. A loving man can contribute by keeping lots of water soluble lubricant or olive oil on hand and sharing plenty of stroking and tenderness before intercourse. (Thirty minutes is not out of line.) Yet once the woman feels relaxed and warmed up, her milk is liable to let-down and squirt all over everything. Humor and understanding will be especially welcome.

This period will not last forever. When ovulation and menstruation start, the vagina will feel moist again, and sexual desire will return.

Further reading

Billings, Evelyn & John:
"*The Billings Method*"
"*Atlas of the Ovulation Method*"

Breastfeeding support groups

La Leche League
listed in your phone book or:
9616 Minneapolis Ave.
P.O. Box 1209
Franklin Park, IL 60131
(312) 455-7730

Nursing Mother's Council
2509 NE Thompson
Portland, OR 97212
(503) 293-0661

Magazines on mothering & breastfeeding

Compleat Mother
Box 399, Mildmay, Ontario
Canada N0G 2J0

Mothering
Box 1690, Santa Fe
New Mexico, 87504

Mother's Underground
Box 34815
Chicago, IL 60634

Patterns for nursing fashions
(for discreet nursing anywhere)
Elizabeth Lee Designs
P.O. Box 696
Bluebell, UT 84007
(send $3 for catalog
& 2 newsletters)

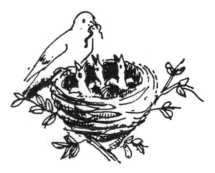

After the Pill

Contraceptive pills prevent a woman's cervix from secreting fertile mucus. Oral contraceptives also stop ovulation most of the time, alter tubal movements so that an egg moves down the fallopian tube too quickly, and they make the uterus hostile to a fertilized egg, should one try to implant.

You can't learn fertility awareness while you are on oral contraceptives because of the overwhelming changes the Pill creates in the reproductive system. But the moment you stop taking contraceptive pills, you can start to regulate your own fertility using natural means.

A few days after you stop taking oral contraceptives, you will have some bleeding or spotting, the same kind of "false period" you had while taking the Pill. Now that you are removing the artificial hormones permanently, three months to a year or two may pass before your body resumes its own natural hormonal functioning. Your temperature and cervical mucus discharges will illustrate how your body is recovering.

Typical mucus patterns after the Pill

Some women have long creamy fertile mucus build-ups, with less than 10 days from the last mucus day until menstruation. A short "post-Peak" phase shows that the body is probably not yet making enough progesterone to support a pregnancy.

Continuous *unchanging* dampness for more than 14 days in a row is a pattern of *infertility*. The sensation at your vulva will feel *dry*. *ANY CHANGE*—more wetness, lubrication, clarity, stretchiness, spotting or bleeding—signals *fertility*.

The mucus may go back and forth between fertile and infertile, then over the months, the pattern will become clearer. *(Please call on a teacher, pp. 136-138, for assistance.)*

A temperature chart can be most useful in confirming when you have finally ovulated. After discontinuing the Pill, some women have experimented with using light to regulate their cycles and clarify the mucus pattern. (*See* page 84.)

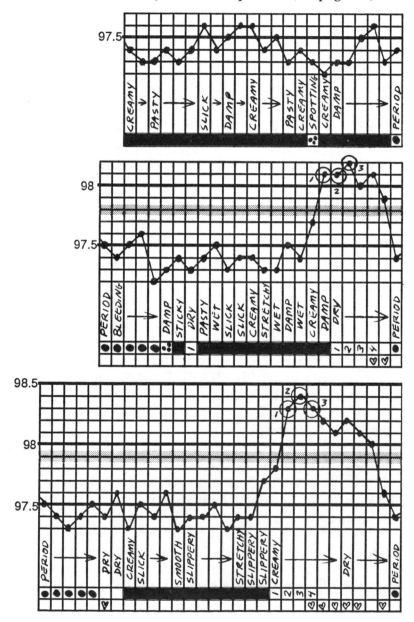

Effects of the Pill

The most well known effect of oral contraceptives is, of course, pregnancy prevention. However, in the process of completely changing your normal hormonal system, the Pill frequently causes other damages. Sometimes these health changes are referred to as "side-effects," as if the only real effect is contraception and the other effects are negligible. For women who experience them, "side-effects" from the Pill are all too real.

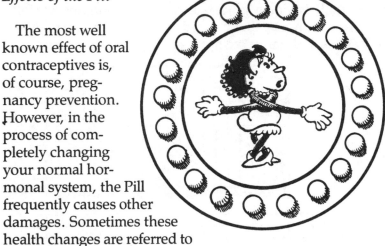

Health risks due to oral contraceptives

Thromboembolism (blood clots), stroke, and hypertension (high blood pressure) are well known effects of oral contraceptives. The new low-dose or triphasic pills lessen these effects. However, the low-dose pills allow more breakthrough bleeding — a signal that ovulation is not being thoroughly suppressed.[1] And that means there's a higher probability of surprise pregnancy.

Women who run the highest risks are those who smoke, and those over 35 years of age. Also at extra risk are those who take the Pill for a long period of time, and women who begin at an early age.

But non-smokers or smokers, women of all ages may gain weight, have headaches, fatigue, vaginal infections, mild to severe depression and wild emotional swings.

Premenstrual syndrome symptoms often become more severe when a woman either starts or stops taking the Pill (p. 57).

Sex drive sometimes decreases when a woman is on the Pill. The Pill can also affect vision.

Some women remain infertile for months or years after they stop taking contraceptive pills.[2] Couples who planned to start their family immediately after stopping oral contraceptives may not be able to carry out their plans.

Even if a woman does resume ovulation soon after Pill usage ends, it is important to wait four to six months afterwards before becoming pregnant. Conception any sooner often results in miscarriage.

Drug and oral contraceptive interactions

Some prescription or over-the-counter drugs lower the effectiveness of oral contraceptives. For example, pregnancies can result among Pill-users who take tetracycline for acne[3] or antibiotics for infections.[4]

Other drugs go through the body faster or slower than usual when the woman takes oral contraceptives. Check with your doctor, or read the *Physician's Desk Reference* at the library, to find out if other drugs you may be taking interact poorly with the Pill, and about the other effects of oral contraceptives.

Natural birth control is a reality

Some say the Pill causes much damage (possibly even breast cancer, at this writing); proponents claim the "side-effects" are slight. In the author's opinion, it's unthinkable to give women things that harm their bodies solely for the sake of providing unlimited access to intercourse.

Regulating Cycles With Light

How does moonlight affect women's cycles? In the 1970's, one woman, Louise Lacey, found literally hundreds of anthropological sources indicating that non-technological cultures worldwide expected women to menstruate at the dark new moon.[1] Since menstruation follows ovulation by about two weeks, such women were most fertile around the time of the bright full moon.

Lacey experimented with nighttime lighting conditions to see if she could simulate the effects of moonlight, and experience the cycle changes documented by other researchers.[2] She and many readers of her book *Lunaception* discovered that by the third or fourth cycle of light regulation, cycles usually shortened to 29-31 days in length. Also, menstruation became shorter and heavier. The mucus pattern grew more distinct instead of creamy and confusing. These changes were a boon to Lacey, since her cycles had been highly erratic after she stopped taking the Pill.

The experimental technique:

Day 1 is the first day of menstruation.
Nights 1-13: Sleep in total darkness. Block out all window and doorway light. Use a red photographic bulb for light if needed during the night.
Nights 14, 15, and 16: Sleep with a dim light on all night. It can be a 15 watt night-light in the wall, a 40-watt bulb in the closet with the door partly closed, or a dim hall light.
During the rest of the cycle, sleep in total darkness again.

Light regulation might be most helpful when cycles are irregular or have long patches of creamy, confusing mucus. (Keeping a regular eating and sleeping pattern and resolving stress also helps cycles stay more steady.)

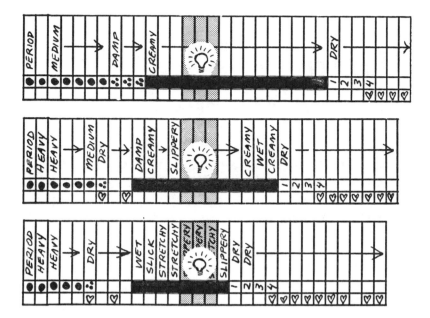

It is thought that sleeping in darkness influences the pineal gland to secrete melatonin, a hormone which inhibits events leading to ovulation. Light at night shuts off melatonin production, so ovulation proceeds.[3]

One historical example

Modern menstrual cycles, under the influence of erratic light at night, do not necessarily correspond to lunar cycles. However, ancient Hebrew customs are evidence of the way one group of people observed a correspondence between their fertility and the lunar cycles. The new moon marked both the beginning of the month, and the time women would celebrate and menstruate together in the desert.[4] Couples refrained from intercourse during menses and for seven days after bleeding ceased. When the separation period was over, around day 12-14 of the cycle, each woman immersed herself in a ritual bath, the *mikveh*. Emerging spiritually and emotionally renewed, she was ready for intercourse again— near her peak of fertility, and probably just as the moon waxed full.

Choosing Your Baby's Sex

Understanding the mucus signals may help a couple select the sex of their baby, according to some ovulation method manuals. One study showed that 310 of 314 couples in Nigeria successfully pre-selected a boy, and 90 of 92 couples successfully pre-selected a girl, using mucus indications.[1]

Naturally choosing a baby's sex is not guaranteed to work. However, the theory is more likely to succeed when the woman has a thorough knowledge of her mucus signs, even though there has been a lot more publicity about using temperature, acid or alkaline douching, and certain lovemaking positions.[2] Temperature alone isn't useful because it only shows when ovulation is finished, and the egg has just a few hours left, if any at all.

The sex pre-selection theory

When one egg cell from the woman unites with a sperm cell from the man, a new life begins. There are two types of sperm cells. Those that cause a boy to be conceived are faster but weaker, while those that cause a girl to be conceived are slower but stronger.[3]

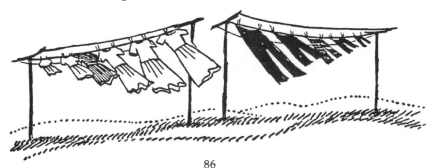

The following guidelines can help couples time intercourse so that mostly the boy-causing or primarily the girl-causing sperm cells are available to unite with the egg.

To have a girl

Make love on the first day of good lubricative mucus. After that, do not make love any more until the evening of the fourth dry day in a row after the last bit of mucus.

The sperm cells will be nourished and waiting for three to five days in the fertile mucus within the cervix. When the egg is finally released, mostly the stronger, girl-causing sperm will still be available. Then they may swim up the fallopian tube to fertilize the egg.

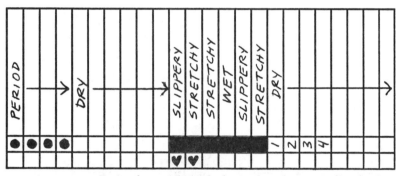

Trying for a girl? Make love when the mucus first begins.

If you do not become pregnant from your first attempt, during the next cycle you might try using the first two days of slippery mucus. After that, you could try the first three days. But you will have a better chance for a girl if you stop making love at least two or more days before you actually ovulate.

Does your temperature start to rise before the mucus is over? Try to stop making love at least two or three days before the temperature rise.

To have a boy

To conceive a boy according to the theory, time intercourse to coincide with ovulation. The faster boy-causing sperm cells will swim up quickly to meet and fertilize the waiting egg, before the slower girl-causing sperm cells can get there.

As soon as fertile mucus begins, avoid intercourse. Since ovulation usually occurs just as the mucus is losing its slippery quality (on the last mucus day, or the day after), make love then, and also on the next one or two dry days.

If you have previously kept three or four accurate charts, you will know how many days of mucus you've been having lately. Then you may guess which is likely to be the final mucus day in the present cycle.

(However, not all of your own cycles will have the same number of mucus days. Fertile phases vary in length and keep sex pre-selection from being fool-proof.)

Hoping for a boy? Make love on the last mucus day and the day or two afterwards.

Low fertility and sex pre-selection

If you want a baby, and your fertile mucus is infrequent or sparse, make love whenever you notice the fertile mucus, and during the next day or two. A woman with very little mucus will not have much control over trying for one sex or the other.

Is it ethical?

Some people maintain that trying to choose the sex of a baby is taking over God's work. Others say that the natural fertility signals are God's gift to us to use as wisely as possible, just as we wisely use the other natural signals such as hunger pangs, sweat, or emotions. At any rate, sex pre-selection cannot be done casually. To improve the couple's chances of success, a woman must observe a few mucus cycles, especially if a boy is desired.

The mucus signal is wonderfully exact when used for fertility control. But mucus varies in small ways, as each woman knows, so that in trying to choose the sex of one's baby, there will always be an element beyond human control.

For the mental health of both mother and baby it is vital to be grateful for the child regardless of its sex.

Does sex pre-selection really work?

Are you curious to find out how effective sex pre-selection might really be? If so, send a copy of the mucus chart showing when you became pregnant, regardless of whether or not you tried to choose the baby's sex. Tell if the baby was born a girl or a boy.

Charts will be checked to see if the girls and boys were consistently conceived from intercourse before, on or after the last mucus day. Enclose a self-addressed stamped envelope so you can receive the results of this inquiry as soon as 100 charts have been tabulated.

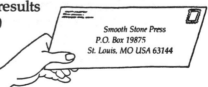

Smooth Stone Press
P.O. Box 19875
St. Louis, MO USA 63144

Menopause
the Natural Way

As they reach the age of 40 or 50, most women will ovulate less frequently and less regularly and mucus production will taper off. Eventually fertility ends altogether.

During pre-menopause, a woman can expect dryness or constant unchanging dampness to gradually replace her wet slippery fertile mucus. Though the fertile mucus will naturally become *less obvious*, the mucus pattern will still show when a woman can or can't get pregnant.

Loving cooperation helps couples avoid pregnancy naturally

With your partner, cooperate in discovering romantic or physical alternatives to intercourse while fertile or unsure of your fertility. Making love when you merely "hope" or "assume" you are infertile may result in an unexpected pregnancy.

When unsure about the fertility signals, some couples use contraceptive barriers instead of natural methods. Usually barriers do prevent pregnancy, although women sometimes get pregnant while using barrier methods during the fertile phase. In addition, spermicides may make it harder to tell when fertile mucus has begun or ended.

Contraceptive pills

Women who take the Pill and are over 35, like those who smoke, run a higher than average risk of heart disease, heart attack, stroke and high blood-pressure. Why should a woman be subject to these dangers when she could use the fertility signals to identify her few remaining fertile days?

90

Becoming pregnant when desired

Women who wish to become pregnant while approaching menopause can use their fertility signals to pinpoint their most fertile days.

Short cycles become more common

Even if you've had long or medium cycles in the past, you may have some very short cycles as you approach menopause.

Follow the usual guidelines

During pre-menopause, follow the usual ovulation method guidelines on pages 16 through 45. Remember that you are fertile when you feel wet and slippery, or have spotting, even if you do not see any pieces of mucus. Fertility continues until the evening of the fourth dry day in a row. You do not need to have regular cycles or "typical" mucus charts; just keep track of your day to day observations of wetness, dryness or spotting.

Unchanging dampness

Continuous *unchanging* dampness for more than 14 days in a row is a pattern of *infertility*. The sensation at your vulva will feel *dry*. *ANY CHANGE*—more wetness, lubrication, clarity, stretchiness, spotting or bleeding—signals *fertility*. *(Please call on a teacher, pp. 136-138, for assistance.)*

Bleeding or spotting

Be especially alert to spotting or bleeding. Unless bleeding or spotting starts 10-16 days after *obvious* fertile mucus, consider the bleeding fertile. Resume intercourse on the evening of the fourth dry day in a row after all bleeding and wetness ends. Temperature will confirm whether or not you have ovulated (page 50).

How effective is the ovulation method during pre-menopause?

In one study by the Drs. John and Evelyn Billings, 97 out of 98 hormonally pre-menopausal women successfully avoided pregnancy for four years. They worked with an ovulation method teacher and were highly motivated to follow the ovulation method guidelines. One couple became pregnant as expected when they knowingly made love on a fertile day.[1]

The author recommends that you seek a teacher's assistance if you are learning about natural fertility control for the first time. Many teachers are listed later in this book.

Signs of decreasing fertility

- Cycles may be irregular, ranging from 17 days to 6 months. You may even menstruate one to two years after what you thought was your final menstrual period.

- The amount of bleeding varies from very light to extremely heavy. You may bleed between periods. If you are bleeding excessively, see your health practitioner.

- Your temperature may continue to rise and fall, indicating ovulation. However, if the cervix does not respond by producing fertile mucus, you will not be fertile. Be watchful, since just a small amount of mucus can help conception happen.

- Menstruation may begin less than 10 days after the mucus Peak, generally indicating an infertile cycle.

- Your temperature may stop rising periodically indicating that you are not ovulating. However, you may continue to menstruate since the uterine lining may build up somewhat even without ovulation.

- Hot flashes may have you alternately putting on and taking off sweaters or blankets throughout the day and night.

Low estrogen levels cause the hot flashes, which generally coincide with dry days.

• Anything you used to notice during your cycles may not happen anymore, for example, bloating, backaches, or abdominal pain *(Mittelschmertz)*, moodiness, and PMS. Breast tenderness may increase or decrease.

• A myriad of emotions may arise when your childbearing years are ending. Talk out your feelings with those closest to you or a counselor.

• Vaginal dryness can cause irritation or painful intercourse. *Self-help suggestions:*
  1) Drink plenty of water — four to eight glasses per day.
  2) Naturally encourage the flow of your own lubricative arousal fluid by sharing 20-60 minutes of relaxed, tender kisses and caresses.

Hysterectomy

The uterus and ovaries are crucial to sexual response, orgasm, and psychological well-being throughout a woman's lifetime. Although doctors may not know this, women do. Of 500 women interviewed by author Naomi Miller Stokes, *"477 (almost 96%) did not care as much for sex after the surgery, and 399 (nearly 80%) lost sexual appetite entirely."* All too often, she found, personality changes, severe depression, suicidal tendencies, and divorce were the legacies of hysterectomy, *especially* when the ovaries had been removed.*

Excessive bleeding will end and fibroids will shrink at menopause. Fibroids may also be treated through wholistic approaches and diet, or removed by myomectomy. Uterine rupture, cancer and tuberculosis do require hysterectomy, but otherwise it is elective surgery, to be chosen or refused by the woman herself. The uterus and ovaries should never be removed *"just in case"* or *"because you don't need them anymore."* After all, would your doctor or husband have his prostate and testicles removed *"just in case"* or because he is finished having children?

For further reading:
The Castrated Woman, What Your Doctor Won't Tell You About Hysterectomy, (Naomi Miller Stokes, Franklin Watts Publ.)
No More Hysterectomies, (Dr. Victoria Hufnagel, New American Library)
Menopause Naturally, Preparing for the Second Half of Life, (Dr. Sadja Greenwood, Volcano Press). Good section on estrogen therapy.

Hormones Trigger the Fertility Signals

Hormones, or natural chemical messengers in the body, control the reproductive cycle and the fertility signals.

When menstruation begins, a woman has low levels of the hormones *estrogen* and *progesterone*. And as menstrual bleeding tapers off, most women will observe dryness at the vaginal opening.

At some point — it may be during menstruation, or hours, weeks, or months after menstruation — the *hypothalamus gland* (at the front of the brain) sends signals to the *pituitary gland* (at the base of the brain) to begin the hormonal events leading to ovulation.

FSH stimulates the follicle-covered eggs to develop

The pituitary gland sends *follicle stimulating hormone* (FSH) to the woman's *ovaries*. Inside each ovary wait hundreds of thousands of immature eggs which were formed before the woman was born. Each egg is enveloped by a *follicle*. FSH stimulates the follicles, and 10-20 eggs begin ripening.

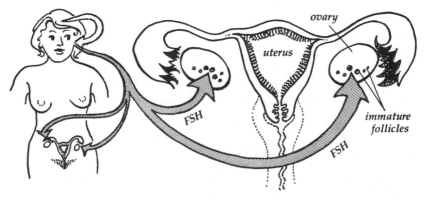

Follicles secrete estrogen,
and estrogen induces mucus production

As they grow, the follicles around the developing eggs secrete estrogen. In response to the estrogen, cave-like crypts inside the cervix secrete wet slippery fertile mucus. Cervical mucus slides downward to the vaginal opening. The mucus signals that eggs are developing and that a woman is fertile.

Estrogen also keeps a woman's basal body temperature relatively low, and causes her cervix to soften, rise up and open slightly. And estrogen stimulates the endometrium (the lining of the uterus) to become enriched with blood, ready to receive a fertilized egg.

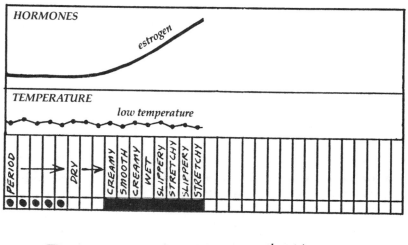

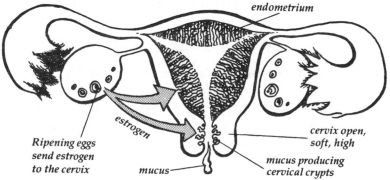

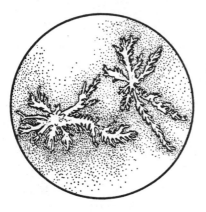

Fertile mucus dried on a glass slide sometimes exhibits a ferning pattern under the microscope.

Rising then falling estrogen levels trigger luteinizing hormone

Near the end of the fertile mucus build-up, the amount of estrogen increases dramatically, then drops, triggering the pituitary gland to release a surge of *luteinizing hormone (LH)* within about 16 hours.

LH causes ovulation on or near the last mucus day

Luteinizing hormone prompts the ripest follicle to burst open, releasing the live egg. Most of the time, ovulation, the release of the live egg, happens on the last day of mucus or the day after.[1]

The two eggs which are released for fraternal twins ovulate within 24 hours of each other.

The fallopian tube sweeps the egg free of the ovary

In a split second, the fringed fimbriae on the end of the fallopian tube reach down and grasp the ovary while the waving of millions of hairlike cilia sucks the egg into the tube.

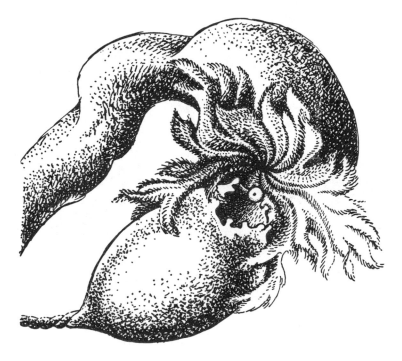

Fallopian tube grasps the ovary and reaches for the ovulated egg.

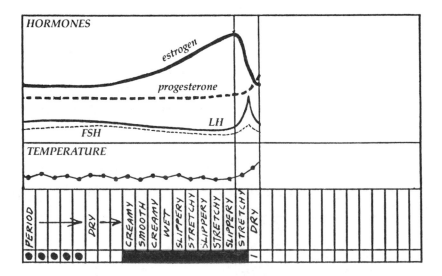

Fertilization and conception

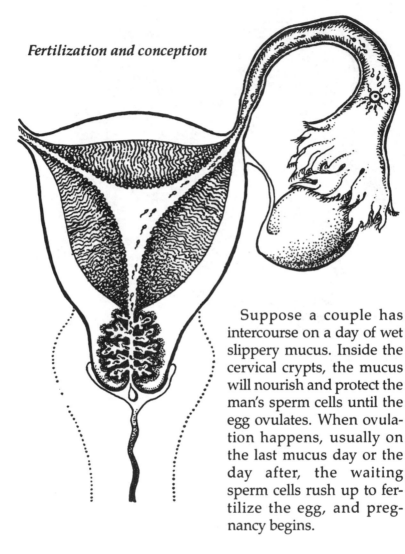

Suppose a couple has intercourse on a day of wet slippery mucus. Inside the cervical crypts, the mucus will nourish and protect the man's sperm cells until the egg ovulates. When ovulation happens, usually on the last mucus day or the day after, the waiting sperm cells rush up to fertilize the egg, and pregnancy begins.

The last mucus day or the day after is the usual time of both ovulation and conception.

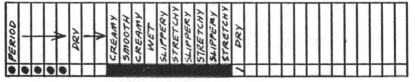

The egg keeps traveling

Muscular contractions and the beating cilia sweep the egg (whether fertilized or not) down the tube towards the uterus

Implantation

A fertilized egg embeds itself within the enriched lining of the uterus. There the embryo grows into a baby, which will be born about 266 days after conception, (give or take six days).

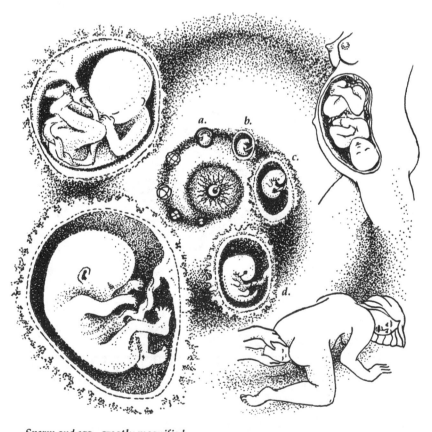

Sperm and egg—greatly magnified.
Actual size: a. 23 days,   b. 28 days,   c. 35 days,   d. 42 days,

Progesterone secreted by the corpus luteum induces dense sticky mucus

After ovulation, the former follicle turns yellow *(luteinizes)* and is called the *corpus luteum* (yellow body). It secretes the hormone *progesterone.*

- Progesterone maintains the blood-filled nutritive lining of the uterus, and keeps a pregnancy going.

- Progesterone also helps raise a woman's basal body temperature.

- And finally, the cervix responds to progesterone by producing dense, sticky *infertile mucus.* Within a few days of ovulation, the infertile mucus prevents sperm from entering the cervix.

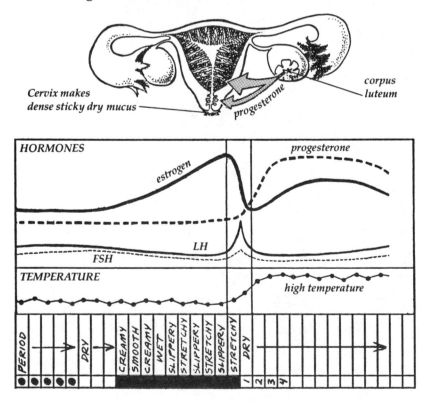

Cervix makes dense sticky dry mucus — progesterone — corpus luteum

Without fertilization the cycle repeats

If there is no fertilized egg, the corpus luteum disintegrates about two weeks after the slippery mucus ends. Lacking progesterone, the uterine lining breaks down and flows out during menstruation. From puberty through menopause, menstruation marks the beginning of a new cycle of fertility and fertility signals.

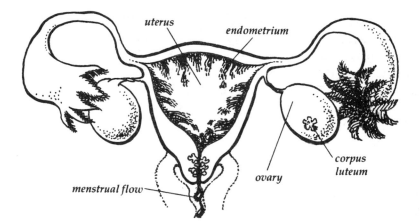

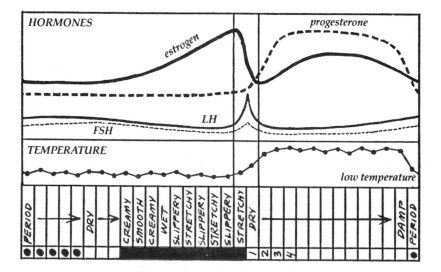

Infertility Self-Help

Understanding the woman's fertility pattern can be the easiest, least stressful, and often the most fruitful step couples can take towards becoming pregnant.

The mucus chart is a valuable tool for physicians and couples. In addition to identifying the fertile phase, fertility signals can help document specific causes of low fertility. The mucus chart can also be used to improve the timing of certain medical tests. Indications on the chart also help couples participate more confidently and actively in the treatments they choose.

Couples who prefer less intervention and ongoing expense will be able to use the fertility signals to identify their most fertile time, even if fertility occurs very rarely for them.

When is a woman most fertile?

Fertility is greatest when a woman has abundant wet, smooth, slippery or stretchy mucus, especially on the last mucus day and the one or two days afterwards. Couples **do not** need to make love on the exact day of ovulation in order to get pregnant. The mucus will keep a man's sperm cells alive inside a woman's body for up to five days, until the egg is released.

Grateful acknowledgement for parts of this chapter go to Suzannah Cooper, author of "Infertility Troubleshooting," (Small World Publications).

Mucus permits sperm cells to continue swimming toward the egg

Fertile cervical mucus is required in order for pregnancy to result from intercourse. Fertile mucus nourishes sperm cells and protects them from the acidic vaginal environment. Long channels in the mucus guide the sperm through the cervix. Without enough fertile mucus, sperm cells are damaged, cannot swim through the cervix, and conception cannot happen.

When does the egg actually ovulate?

About 85% of the time a woman will ovulate on the last day of mucus, or the day after. Another 10% of the time, ovulation takes place from two days before to two days after the last mucus day. After ovulation, the egg lives and can be fertilized for about 12-24 hours.

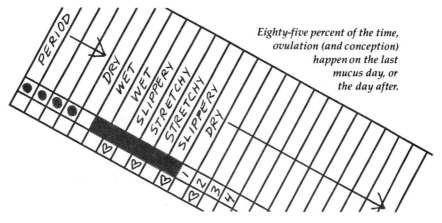

Eighty-five percent of the time, ovulation (and conception) happen on the last mucus day, or the day after.

Ovulation detection kits

Since the easy-to-find mucus accurately pinpoints fertility and ovulation, the mucus signal is, in many cases, a sensible substitute for expensive or uncertain LH detection kits.

Outline for infertility self-help

1. Make love during days or nights of wet, smooth, slippery or stretchy mucus, especially on the last day of mucus, *and* on the first one or two days *after the mucus ends*. The more mucus, the better.

Avoid a marathon. Having intercourse many days in a row can lower the sperm count, making conception more difficult. A 40-48 hour wait lets the man's sperm count increase.

Allow enough time. Couples of normal fertility should expect to make love during the fertile phases of one to six *or more* cycles before becoming pregnant.

2. Temperature tells only when ovulation is over and the egg has little or no time left. If your temperature starts to rise after the mucus ends, it's a reminder to make love after the mucus ends too.[1]

3. Compare your mucus/temperature charts with the charts in this chapter. If you ovulate only once every few months or years, the mucus will alert you to your rare fertile phases. Self-help suggestions are offered for improvement in overall health and fertility.

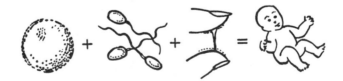

4. A sperm count and semen analysis for the man, and a post-coital test for the couple may be done after about six cycles, or sooner if preferred. Complete these simple tests to your satisfaction before starting any other tests or treatment.

5. After six or more cycles, a couple might choose further medical investigation. Check your doctor's credentials and reputation very carefully. "Infertility specialist" is not a recognized medical specialty in the USA, and any doctor may claim the title, whether qualified or not.[2]

6. Which options best suit your values, relationship and finances: letting nature take its course, medical options, adoption, foster parenting, or remaining childless? Deciding is usually an ongoing process for couples of low fertility. Set aside time to review and possibly revise your decision every few months or years.

7. Resources such as counseling, books, or a Resolve Infertility Support Group may be helpful. To locate a Resolve group in your area, write to RESOLVE, Inc., 5 Water Street, Arlington, MA 02174.

MEN'S INFERTILITY

The man's semen is tested first

The simplest, least expensive and least intrusive fertility tests show whether the man's sperm cells are healthy and numerous. *These tests should always be done before a woman consents to any complex and expensive testing or surgery.*

Semen analysis and sperm count

A semen analysis studies the quantity and quality of the man's sperm cells. If there are not many sperm cells, the man should wait 40-48 hours before ejaculating, to allow his sperm count to increase. White blood cells in the semen may indicate an infection. Some men even produce antibodies to their own sperm, especially if they've had a vasectomy. A large number of dead sperm cells is a clue that there may be sperm antibodies.

Causes of sperm problems

Toxic chemicals, excess heat, or illness can cause deformed or low numbers of sperm. Removing the problem usually allows the generation of new healthier sperm. Sperm cells require about three months to fully mature, so look for improved sperm quality and quantity about three months after eliminating the heat, toxin, or illness. Please turn to page 127 for a list of toxic substances.

Excessive testicular heat

Excessive heat results from anything that pushes the testicles against the body, such as wearing tight underwear or pants, being overweight, sitting for long periods of time (truck driving, desk jobs, long distance bike riding, etc.) Work around hot furnaces or ovens may also be too hot for good sperm production, as can hot-tubbing. An illness with a high fever may also lower a man's sperm count.

A man might consider being transferred to a cooler section of the workplace, or even changing jobs.

There are also a few types of *testicular cooling devices*, for men who cannot avoid heat. Ask your doctor about them.

No sperm at all

A man can have a normal sex drive, erection and ejaculation, but still may not have sperm cells in his seminal fluid. This may be due to reproductive organ damage which will require medical assistance to identify and overcome.

For further reading

Dr. Mark Perloe's book *Miracle Babies*, (Penguin Books) includes a thorough section on men's infertility.

Post-coital test

Within two to three hours of lovemaking *on a day of slippery fertile mucus*, the doctor will examine a sample of the mucus and sperm. He or she can then see if there are live sperm swimming vigorously through the mucus. The test will be inaccurate if done when there is no mucus.

Semen analysis normal; no sperm at all in the post coital test.

The man is not ejaculating inside of his partner. For pregnancy to happen, the couple must place semen in the fertile mucus inside the vagina or on the vaginal lips.

Semen analysis normal; post-coital test shows quivering or immobilized sperm

Artificial ingredients. Douches, sprays, and spermicidal foams, cream or jelly will all immobilize and damage sperm cells. The infertile mucus produced after ovulation also damages sperm cells and blocks them from the cervix.

Sperm-mucus interaction. There may be a problem interaction between the woman's mucus and the man's sperm. In many cases, pregnancy results without any intervention.[3] Tests will show if the mucus/sperm interaction is limited to the two partners, or if the mucus is hostile to sperm from other donors too.

Some couples experiment with naturally reducing the woman's sperm antibodies. The couple uses condoms, and makes sure that no semen touches the woman anywhere, (on skin, mouth, vagina, etc.), for about six months.

Semen analysis normal;
white blood cells in the post-coital sample

The woman may have an infection such as mycoplasma urea or chlamydia. These or other infections can prevent conception, and may be treated with antibiotics. Vaginal infections can also make conception difficult. Both partners must be treated in order to stop spreading a vaginal infection back and forth to each other. (See the *Vaginal Infections* chapter.)

Timing of women's infertility tests

The *progesterone blood level* should be drawn on days five, seven and nine after the last mucus day, to give a baseline reading. In subsequent cycles, the blood can be taken on day seven after the mucus ends. An *endometrial biopsy* can easily be scheduled one or two days before menstruation by referring back to previous mucus charts.[4] Menstruation often begins the same number of days after the mucus ends for an individual woman.

On the next few pages you'll find mucus and temperature charts with some (not all) of the possible corresponding infertility problems. Simpler situations, many arising from fertility *un*awareness, are listed first for each chart. **Beginning on page 116 an alphabetical list describes each situation in more detail.**

This book emphasizes self-help, so for medical opinions, diagnoses or treatment, consult your doctor.

Your own basal body temperature may be far higher or lower than the temperatures depicted in this book.

A. Normal mucus and temperature

Teresa's mucus and temperature patterns indicate ovulation and normally cycling reproductive hormones. She is fertile on any day of mucus, especially the last mucus day and the one or two days after the mucus ends.

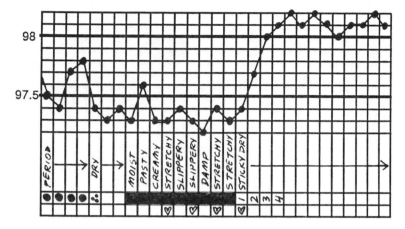

Normal mucus and temperature
Possible factors

take enough time
semen analysis
sperm count tested
post-coital test needed
douching
artificial lubricants
spermicides
vaginal infection
bladder infection
other minor infections
sexual technique
too much sex
I.U.D.
too much exercise
toxic substances
   cigarette smoke

prescription
   or "recreational" drugs
diet
weight
stress
sperm-mucus interaction
kidney and liver diseases
uterine problems
D.E.S. exposure
vasectomy
adhesions
endometriosis
pelvic inflammatory disease
uterine problems
tubal problems
tubal ligation

More details begin on page 116.

B. Last low temperature after the Peak day...

There was not much mucus available to protect the sperm after Joanne's mucus ended, even though she might have been ovulating then. So the couple made love on the dry days after the mucus ended, in addition to using a few wet mucus days.

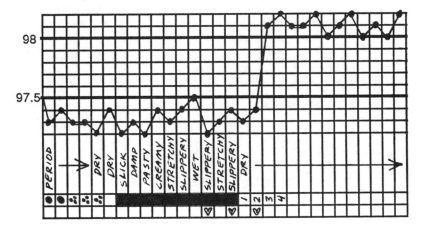

C. Last low temperature before the Peak day...

...may indicate that Sue ovulated before her mucus ended. She and her partner made sure they had intercourse on the wet mucus days before the temperature rose, as well as afterwards.

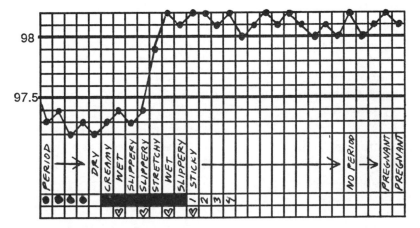

D. Short cycles

Judy might have ovulated on day 5, her last day of wet slippery mucus, or on the next day. Her consistently high temperature and lack of menstruation 17 days later confirmed her pregnancy (unless high temperature was due to fever).

Sometimes women are told they will ovulate around the fourteenth day of their cycle. This is an outdated Rhythm method myth. Ovulation can and does occur *any* number of days after menstruation begins, and is predicted by wet, slippery cervical mucus.

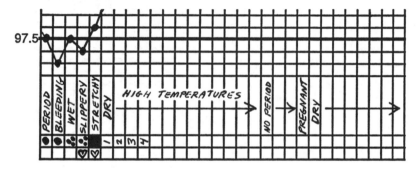

E. Delayed ovulation

Stress caused Sonia's wet but confusing mucus to taper off, then to begin again more clearly later on (see page 38). She probably ovulated on day 18, the last mucus day, or the day after. If she is not pregnant, her period will begin about two weeks later.

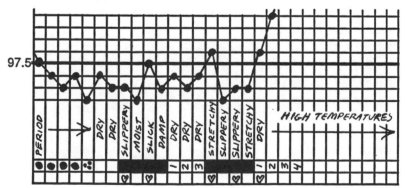

F. Short luteal phase

Menstruation began less than 10 days after Corinna's fertile mucus ended. In this cycle, her corpus luteum (formerly the follicle surrounding the ripening egg) probably did not make enough progesterone to support a pregnancy.

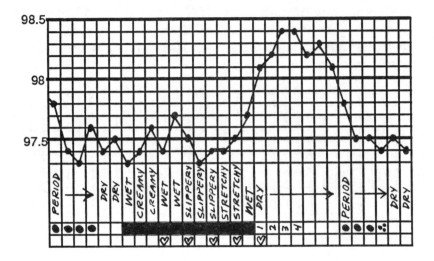

Short luteal phase
Possible factors involved

breastfeeding
exercise (too much)
diet
the Pill
prolactin level, elevated
thyroid problems
pre-menopause
D.E.S. exposure
(men's infertility)

More details begin on page 116.

G. No mucus, normal temperature

The rising temperature chart shows that Laura is ovulating. Either she isn't finding the mucus, or her cervix is not responding to estrogen by making fertile mucus. Mucus is necessary for conception because it protects the sperm from the acidic vagina, permits the sperm to enter the cervix and uterus, and nourishes the sperm until ovulation.

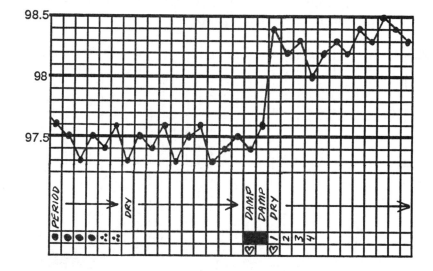

No mucus, normal temperatures
Possible factors

finding the mucus	vaginal infections
creamy mucus	oral contraceptives
swimming	thyroid problems
infrequent mucus	pre-menopause
diet	D.E.S. exposure
antihistamines	conization of cervix
douching	other damage to cervix
lubricants	hysterectomy
spermicides	(men's infertility)

More details begin on page 116.

H. Constant or intermittent mucus, no temperature change

Estrogen is stimulating Tanya's cervix, but her temperature shows that she is not ovulating.

It's normal to skip ovulation once in a while. And during breastfeeding, a woman may have weeks or months of constantly changing wet mucus without ovulation. But for a non-breastfeeding woman, such a pattern may point to excess estrogen and hormonal feedback problems.

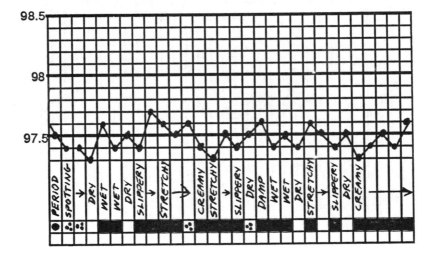

Constant or intermittent mucus, no temperature change
Some factors involved

occasional anovulatory cycle
broken thermometer
review temperature method
breastfeeding
stress
obesity
irritated or damaged cervix
    (may cause constant discharge)

contraceptive Pill
thyroid problems
liver or kidney problems
D.E.S. exposure
polycystic ovaries
rare ovulation
(men's infertility)

More details begin on page 116.

I. No mucus, no temperature rise.

The temperature shows that Debbie did not ovulate during this cycle. There may be all kinds of reasons why — hormonal, physical, emotional, environmental, or others. Women normally have occasional anovulatory cycles, but since Debbie almost never ovulates, she stays aware of her mucus in order to spot her rare fertile phases.

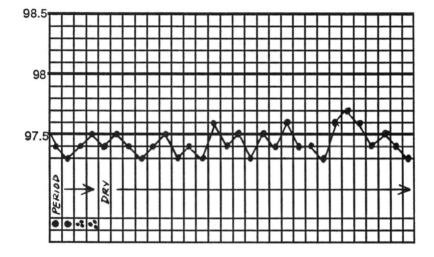

No mucus, no temperature rise.
Possible factors involved

the Pill	thyroid problems
breastfeeding	rare ovulation
diet	prolactin level (elevated)
weight	menopause
exercise	pituitary or other
stress	hormonal problems
pre-menopause	polycystic ovaries
toxic substances	ovarian problems
drugs, prescription	hysterectomy
or "recreational"	(men's infertility)
pelvic inflammatory disease	

More details begin on page 116.

Alphabetical listing of some common infertility problems

ADHESIONS (scar tissue) around the tubes, uterus, and/or ovaries can immobilize your organs and prevent pregnancy. Scar tissue commonly results from abdominal surgery, gonorrhea or other pelvic inflammatory diseases, or a ruptured appendix. Sometimes adhesions can be removed surgically, although they may grow back.

ADRENAL GLAND ABNORMALITIES produce elevated androgen (male hormone) levels. An overweight woman's fat cells may convert the androgen to excess estrogen. Constant or intermittent fertile-type mucus may result. Psychological or physical stresses sometimes help cause adrenal diseases.

ANTIHISTAMINES will dry up cervical mucus along with clearing your sinuses.

BLADDER INFECTIONS are so painful that a woman will not be interested in sex. Spermicidal foam, jelly, etc. are common causes. *Self-help suggestion to alleviate pain:* when you first notice frequent brief urination, immediately drink ½ teaspoon baking soda dissolved in a cup of cold water, every ½ hour for 2 hours. Repeat once per hour for 2-4 hours. And see your physician as soon as possible.

BREASTFEEDING. The hormone *prolactin* is released in response to the baby sucking on the mother's breast. Prolactin stimulates milk production, but generally hinders ovulation. As breastfeeding tapers off, prolactin levels drop, and ovulation and cycling resume. The luteal phase may be short during the first few cycles after breastfeeding because the prolactin level might still be higher than usual. During breastfeeding, the temperature and mucus pattern will not cycle until the woman ovulates again. In the meantime, she will have dryness, patches of fertile appearing mucus or spotting, or constant mucus.

CERVICAL DAMAGE due to disease, D.E.S. exposure, or surgery can cause constantly changing creamy or gummy mucus, or no mucus at all.

CONIZATION OF THE CERVIX. A cone shaped slice of tissue is cut out of the cervix, sometimes in response to continuous discharges, or finding abnormal or precancerous cells. Once conization removes your cervical crypts, they are gone forever, 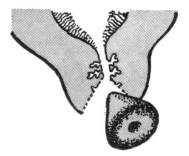 along with your mucus producing capability and fertility. If some crypts remain, you will still have mucus, but less than usual. It may be harder to spot fertility both to get pregnant and to prevent pregnancy naturally.

The cervix is weakened by conization. An *"incompetent cervix"* can suddenly open up during pregnancy, letting a growing baby slip out prematurely.

Seek a second or third doctor's opinion before consenting to conization of your cervix.

CRYOSURGERY OR ELECTROCAUTERY electrically freezes or burns a portion of the cervix, sometimes in order to combat abnormal cells or constant harmless discharges. Mucus producing cervical crypts may be damaged, although the crypts may grow back. Application of silver nitrate is a much gentler alternative than cryosurgery, cauterization, or conization.[5]

D.E.S. DAUGHTERS were in the womb when their mothers took the drug diethylstilbestrol, under the false assumption that it would prevent miscarriages. The drug was in use from 1941-1971 in the United States, then it was banned for human consumption.

D.E.S. sons and daughters frequently developed

reproductive and hormonal abnormalities as they reached adolescence.

One common problem is a **cervical eversion or ectropian** ("inside out" cervix) which may result in **constant discharges**. Silver nitrate application is a gentler and less invasive treatment than cryosurgery, cauterization, or the fertility-diminishing cone biopsy (see above). D.E.S.-caused ectropians usually heal naturally by the age of about 30.[6] **Gummy mucus discharges, cyclic recurrent bleeding,** and **unusual or pre-cancerous cervical cells** are also common to D.E.S. daughters. Charting cyclic bleeding and discharges allows a woman to avoid unnecessary treatment.

D.E.S. daughters often experience **long, creamy fertile mucus** build-ups followed by a frustratingly **short luteal phase**. This type of mucus pattern is typical of **hormonal problems.**[7]

For more information contact D.E.S. Action, 2845 24th St., San Francisco, CA 94110, phone (415) 826-5060, or D.E.S. Action offices in New Hyde Park, N.Y., Montreal, Quebec, or Camberwell, Victoria, Australia.

DIET, WEIGHT & EXERCISE. Normally, fat helps to store a woman's estrogen until enough of the hormone builds up to help trigger ovulation. However, a woman with **less than the optimum 15-20% body fat** may "burn-up" her estrogen supply before it reaches a peak which will allow ovulation. As a result, many runners, ballet dancers, some vegetarians, anorexic women and others stop ovulating and cycling. Self-help approaches to restoring fertility include:

1. Gradually reducing exercise until cycling resumes.

2. Temporarily gaining 5 to 10 pounds in order to optimize the chances of ovulating. The extra weight may be shed later on.

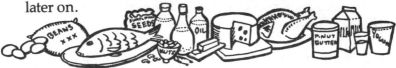

3. Eating more unprocessed, unsaturated vegetable oils, fats and proteins which are the building blocks of reproductive hormones. Also add the essential mineral zinc (from raw pumpkin seeds).

Sometimes a woman may **increase the mucus flow** by taking normal amounts of vitamin B$_6$.

Getting pregnant is difficult for some **overweight women**. Normally, estrogen levels drop before menstruation, signaling that conception did not occur. But excess fat stores and releases estrogen at constant, moderately high levels. Without the low-estrogen signal, the brain is sluggish about stimulating egg development in the next cycle. The result? Continuous or intermittent slippery mucus, very long irregular cycles, or overly heavy periods.

In one study, losing weight on a healthy diet helped 11 out of 13 patients start ovulating again, and 10 conceived. (Average weight dropped from 169 to 149 pounds.)[8] On the other hand, the stress of crash diets or sudden overly rigorous exercise can delay ovulation instead of enhancing fertility.

Apparently, sudden weight gain is more apt to disrupt the cycle than weight an ovulating woman has carried for years.

DOUCHING washes away some of the cervical mucus and makes it hard to find for a few hours. Douching also changes the pH (acid/alkaline balance) of the vagina, encourages vaginal infections, and weakens sperm cells. The vagina is self-cleansing, and regular douching is not recommended. To safely remedy an itchy, smelly vaginal infection, turn to the *"Vaginal Infections"* chapter.

ENDOMETRIOSIS. When a woman has endometriosis bits of endometrial tissue, the kind that normally lines the uterus, are found scattered throughout her abdomen. During the cycle the stray tissue swells with blood, like the normal uterine lining does. At menstruation the scattered endometrial tissue bleeds too, causing severe pain. Sometimes the pain subsides the longer a woman has endometriosis.

Surgical and hormonal treatments have been tried with varying degrees of success. *For more information, phone 1-800-992-ENDO or read "Overcoming Endometriosis, New Help From the Endometriosis Association", by Mary Lou Ballweg & the Endometriosis Assoc., Box 92187, Milwaukee, WI 53202 ($9.95).*

FINDING THE MUCUS. Fertile mucus may be present only once during a fertile day. That's why it is important to check for mucus by wiping the vaginal opening before and after each use of the toilet (p. 24). You are considered fertile even if you merely *feel* wet and slippery as you wipe. You may not see any mucus. Or, wiping may feel dry though you do see some mucus.

Also be alert throughout the day to a wet feeling similar to that of menstruation. Your fertile mucus could be sliding down. And be sensitive to the suddenly increasing energy, emotional excitement and sexual desire which often signal fertility.

Swimming may wash away external mucus temporarily. Check internally for mucus during the day, and at night do the Kegel exercise: contract and relax your muscles a few times as if stopping and starting the flow of urine. Then bear down, and observe your mucus.

Wet creamy mucus is fertile too. The mucus need not stretch. If you merely feel smooth slippery wetness, you are potentially fertile.

Not much mucus. You may ovulate and have wet fertile mucus only once in many months or years. The mucus will show you the fertile time.

HORMONAL PROBLEMS. A prolonged, confusing creamy mucus build-up followed by a short post-ovulatory phase commonly reflects hormonal problems. Such a pattern is typical after stopping **oral contraceptives**, or in a woman exposed to **D.E.S.** before birth. Cycles usually normalize a few months to a few years after a woman stops taking the Pill. Some former Pill users have used light to help regulate cycles and clarify the mucus pattern. (*see* Pill)

HYSTERECTOMY, or removal of the uterus and cervix lowers the chances of pregnancy to nearly zero. Of course if the cervix is gone, a woman will not have fertile mucus.

Hysterectomy is required only for uterine cancer, rupture, or tuberculosis. It will end the pain of endometriosis. But there are other ways of treating fibroids which leave the uterus intact. Since removal of the uterus, (and especially removal of ovaries) diminishes sexual desire and induces depression and relationship problems, seek the alternatives. Read: *The Castrated Woman, What Your Doctor Won't Tell You About Hysterectomy*, (N. Stokes), and *No More Hysterectomies*, (V. Hufnagel).

INFECTIONS. *see* Pelvic Inflammatory Diseases, and Vaginal Infections.

I.U.D. If you thought you "lost" an intra-uterine device, have another health practitioner check to see if you only lost the string. The I.U.D. may still be inside you, preventing pregnancy. Also, the string on an I.U.D. can conduct infectious bacteria into the uterus, resulting in infertility. *see* Pelvic Inflammatory Disease.

KIDNEY AND LIVER DISEASES prevent filtration of toxins and hormones from the bloodstream. Estrogen and other hormones can accumulate, interfering with egg development, ovulation, and cycling. In addition to medical treatment, reduce the workload of your liver and kidneys: avoid eating preservatives, colorings, additives or pesticides, and eat more whole unrefined, unprocessed foods.

LIGHT, effect on cycles. *see* Pill

LUTEAL PHASE PROBLEMS. A short luteal phase means less than 10 days from the last fertile mucus until the beginning of menstruation. A short post-ovulatory phase shows that the corpus luteum (formerly the follicle) is probably not secreting enough progesterone to support the uterine lining or a pregnancy.

Sometimes progesterone suppositories supply the needed hormone, and treatment begins soon after ovulation. Ovulation is signaled naturally as the fertile mucus loses its slippery quality, on the last mucus day or the day after. Progesterone treatment continues until the baby's placenta produces enough progesterone to maintain pregnancy.

MENOPAUSE, PRE-MENOPAUSE. Irregular cycles and mucus which is less obvious than usual are normal during pre-menopause. However, wetness, lubrication, spotting or stretchy mucus still indicate potential fertility. Heightened sexual desire, energy and excitement may also alert a woman to increasing fertility. Temperature will confirm ovulation.

MEN'S INFERTILITY. Either or both partners may have infertility problems. Some of those affecting men are described at the beginning of this chapter.

OVARIAN PROBLEMS. Unusual spotting or mucus patterns sometimes signal ovarian problems. **Cysts, tumors, or endometriosis** may respond to medical treatment. **Infections** can stop ovulation and mucus production, and may also cause blocked tubes or scarring which further impair fertility. After **radiation**, perhaps for a tumor, any healthy ovarian tissue remaining may heal and eventually produce viable eggs again.

High FSH (follicle-stimulating hormone) levels may indicate **premature ovarian failure** (early menopause) as the pituitary keeps trying to stimulate non-functioning ovaries.

Polycystic ovaries do not ovulate despite constantly high LH (luteinizing hormone) levels. The fat cells of an overweight woman with this condition will manufacture excess estrogen from androgens which build up in the ovary. The estrogen may cause constant or intermittent fertile-type mucus.

If the ovaries are **completely destroyed by radiation**, or are **removed surgically**, the woman may become depressed, and will have little or no interest in sex, the same as a man whose testicles have been removed. In addition, she will be dependent upon estrogen treatments, and of course will not cycle or have mucus and temperature changes. *(See page 93.)*

PELVIC INFLAMMATORY DISEASE (PID). Sexually transmitted diseases such as chlamydia, gonorrhea, syphilis and others, can cause painful abdominal infections which result in damaged, scarred immobilized reproductive organs, blocked tubes, and infertility. Some signs of PID are severe abdominal pain, fever, and white blood cells in the mucus. PID must be immediately treated with antibiotics.

Avoiding multiple sex partners lowers the risk of catching PID. Also, avoid wearing an I.U.D. The string wicks harmful bacteria up into the uterus, causing severe infections and often sterility.

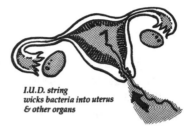

I.U.D. string wicks bacteria into uterus & other organs

PILL. Contraceptive pills usually (though not always) prevent pregnancy when taken according to instructions. While taking the Pill, a woman will not have cyclic fertile mucus or temperature patterns. Miscarriages are common if a woman becomes pregnant sooner than four to six months after she stops taking oral contraceptives.

When she stops taking the Pill, a woman may have three months to a few years of cycles with long phases of creamy wetness instead of short patches of obviously fertile mucus. In addition, menstruation may begin less than 10 days after the mucus ends. These cycles show that the woman's hormonal system is still in the process of healing and is not yet functioning normally.

Some women experiment with **using light** to help the *pineal gland* regulate their cycles and boost recovery. The woman simply sleeps in absolute darkness except on the 14th, 15th and 16th days after menstruation begins. On those nights, she leaves a small light bulb on in the room. After two or three cycles, many women find that their mucus pattern is more distinct, menstruation is shorter and heavier, and cycles become 29-31 days in length.[9]

POLYCYSTIC OVARIES. *see* Ovarian Problems.

PREGNANCY. A pregnant woman will not have fertile mucus nor cyclic temperature changes. Her steady high temperature shows that she is not ovulating, and if she bleeds lightly, the consistently high temperature keeps confirming pregnancy. Her mucus will be sticky and dense.

Natural signs of pregnancy: No menstruation 14-17 days after obviously fertile mucus ends; and a high temperature (not a fever) for 17 or more days in a row after fertile mucus is over.

PRE-MENOPAUSE. *see* Menopause.

PROLACTIN LEVEL, elevated. Prolactin is the hormone which naturally hinders ovulation while a woman is breast-feeding. Sometimes other medical problems or drugs will elevate the prolactin level and keep a non-breastfeeding woman from becoming pregnant or staying pregnant. One of the external signs of a high prolactin level is a milky discharge from the breasts. *See also* Breastfeeding.

Possible medical problems: pituitary tumor, too much stress or exercise, kidney disease, low thyroid, adrenal disease, polycystic ovaries. *Some medications which may cause a high prolactin level:* methyldopa (aldomet), narcotics, reserpine, phenothiazines, tranquilizers, tricyclic antidepressants.[10]

RADIATION. *see* Men's Infertility, and Ovarian Problems.

RARE OVULATION. Some women only ovulate once every few months or years. Fertile mucus will signal potential fertility. *see* Finding the Mucus.

RUNNING. *see* Exercise

SEXUAL TECHNIQUE. In order for pregnancy to result from intercourse, sperm must reach the cervix during the fertile phase, or at least get into fertile mucus in the vagina or on the vaginal lips. Once the sperm cells land in the mucus, they can swim up the mucus channels to the cervix and onward to the egg.

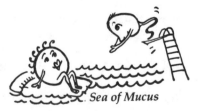

Sea of Mucus

Getting the sperm to the mucus. If the man doesn't ejaculate, a few drops of sperm-rich pre-ejaculatory fluid could be placed on the mucus at the vaginal opening.

Insemination. If the man ejaculates outside of the woman, the couple could collect the seminal fluid and squirt it near the cervix using a plastic gravy baster from the kitchen. Gently place the semen in the vagina (*not* inside the cervix itself.) Fertile mucus will allow the sperm cells to swim through the cervix. The mucus will filter out the seminal liquid which is highly toxic if it enters the uterus.

Too much sex. Make love on alternate days or nights while fertile, or even less frequently, to allow at least 40-48 hours for the man's sperm count to increase.

When to have intercourse. The last mucus day and the day or two after are the most fertile of all, though every mucus day is potentially fertile.

SPERM-MUCUS INTERACTION. Sometimes the man's sperm and the woman's mucus are not compatible, although the couple may become pregnant anyway. Antibodies in the woman's mucus can attack her partner's sperm cells. To experiment with naturally reducing the woman's sperm antibodies, the couple may use condoms, and avoid all contact between the woman's skin, mouth, vagina, etc. and the semen for three to six months.

SPERMICIDAL FOAMS, JELLIES, CREAMS, LUBRI-CANTS, etc. are meant to kill sperm cells and prevent pregnancy. Spermicides may also mask fertile mucus for about a day after their use, and can cause painful bladder infections.

STRESS affects the hypothalamus, a gland which is very sensitive to emotions, exercise, diet, light, etc. As a result of stress, the hypothalamus may interrupt hormonal messages which lead to ovulation. Travel, illness, worry and excitement are just a few of the stresses which may cause you to ovulate earlier than usual, or delay ovulation for days, weeks, or longer. Even while under stress, the mucus will signal your fertility day by day, although it may take more patience than usual to wait until you are sure you are fertile.

Self-help approaches to dealing with stress include daily exercise, cutting down on sugar, caffeine and refined foods, seeking counseling, doing relaxation exercises and stretching, and repeating affirmations.

Affirmations are sentences with emotional words describing how you would actually feel as you accomplish your desires. For instance, *"I'm beautifully radiating glowing health."* As you repeat the affirmations before bedtime, vividly see, feel, and hear yourself in the situation you describe. Affirmations provide a powerful way of talking yourself into reducing stress, improving your health, feeling energetic and successfully accomplishing your goals.[11]

SWIMMING. *see* Finding the Mucus.

TAKE ENOUGH TIME. Even couples of normal fertility may make love during the fertile phases of at least six cycles before becoming pregnant.

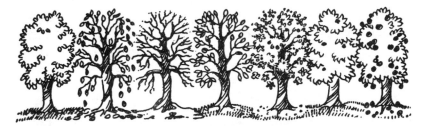

TECHNOLOGICAL APPROACHES. There are technologies which allow eggs to be fertilized through means other than intercourse, although they are beyond the scope of this book. A library, bookstore, family planning center or physician can provide more information on these processes. Nobody knows for sure how these processes will affect the baby or its descendants.

TEMPERATURE METHOD. You can begin taking your temperature when the mucus starts. Take your temperature each morning before moving around, eating or smoking. Check that your thermometer is not broken. Remember, the temperature chart shows when ovulation is *finished*. To predict ovulation in advance, and to know exactly when you are fertile, observe your mucus. *(Temperature directions begin on page 46.)*

THYROID PROBLEMS. Too much thyroid increases the metabolism. A woman with **hyperthyroidism** will use up estrogen before it reaches a high enough level to trigger luteinizing hormone and ovulation. Without enough estrogen, she may not have much fertile mucus either. **Hypothyroidism**, or low thyroid, slows the metabolism, so estrogen builds up in the bloodstream instead of being removed as required. The chart will show many unusually low temperature readings, and an excessive number of mucus days. *(Reading: "Hypothyroidism, the Unsuspected Illness," Barnes.)*

TESTICULAR HEAT from tight underwear, obesity, prolonged sitting, a hot workplace, hot-tubbing, or fever can lower a man's sperm count. The count should improve about three months after the heat ends. *See* Men's Infertility.

TOXIC SUBSTANCES at home or at the workplace, can interfere with both men's and women's fertility. Potentially harmful substances include alcohol, caffeine, some drugs (both prescription and "recreational"), cigarette smoke, marijuana, radiation, and chemicals such as lead, organic solvents, pesticides, polystyrene, benzene, mercury, anesthetic gases, and Agent Orange. Fertility usually improves after exposure stops, unless the damage is already too severe. Ways to avoid toxic substances include wearing protective gloves, masks, or clothing, transferring to a different department, changing jobs altogether, or moving to a different house or neighborhood.

TUBAL PROBLEMS. If you had your **tubes "tied"** for permanent birth control, or if the tubes were cut accidentally due to other surgery or an injury, the fertilized egg will usually be unable to travel to the uterus. The chances of pregnancy are lowered to about 1% *(also PMS symptoms and menstrual cramps may worsen)*.

Scar tissue from surgery or pelvic inflammatory disease can immobilize or block the tubes and prevent pregnancy.

Blocked tubes. The tubes are not smooth and hollow, like a garden hose. It doesn't take much obstruction to keep sperm and egg from traveling freely through the tubes.

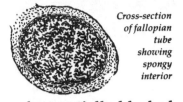

Cross-section of fallopian tube showing spongy interior

Tiny sperm may swim up through a **partially blocked** tube and can unite with the egg. On its way back down the tube, the large fertilized egg may become trapped. The **tubal or ectopic pregnancy** that develops in the tube becomes extremely painful and threatens the life of the mother. The pregnancy usually must be surgically removed.

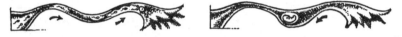

Sexually transmitted diseases, and infections due to I.U.D.s are the primary causes of tubal problems. To reduce your risks, avoid I.U.D.s and multiple sex partners, and make sure your partner does not have a sexually transmitted disease in the first place. (*see* Adhesions, Pelvic Inflammatory Disease)

UTERINE PROBLEMS. Infection, abdominal surgery, a vigorous abortion, or an I.U.D. can cause **adhesions or scarring** inside the uterus. Endometrial growth, egg implantation and fetal growth can be hindered, and infertility or miscarriage may occur. Sometimes minor surgery is helpful.

Fibroids are growths which may interfere with fertility. They may be removed by *myomectomy*, or diminished through wholistic and dietary approaches. *Hysterectomy* (removal of the uterus) is unnecessary (see page 93).

D.E.S. exposure while a baby girl was in her mother's womb may have resulted in a T-shaped, divided, or undersized uterus once the girl matured. (*see* D.E.S.)

The uterus can take a variety of unusual shapes, sizes and positions. Many a woman with an unusually shaped uterus conceives and carries a baby to term. Each case is individual.

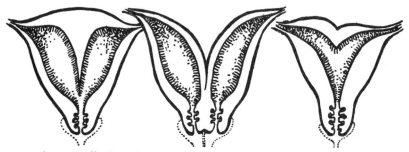

An unusually shaped uterus may or may not interfere with fertility.

VAGINAL INFECTIONS interfere with fertility by impeding sperm movement. Some suggestions for clearing up vaginitis are described in the *"Vaginal Infections"* chapter.

VASECTOMY. A man with a vasectomy has had his vas deferens cut, so that sperm cells cannot leave his body when he ejaculates. As a result, he cannot father children. He may, in fact, start producing antibodies against the billions of sperm cells which have accumulated inside him. Sometimes vasectomy reversals are successful, although antibodies may still interfere with fertility.

A closing word

Couples trying hard to become pregnant often turn lovemaking into a pressured, frustrating chore. By understanding when to expect infertility as part of the normal cycle, the beloveds can choose to share intercourse attentively with each other, instead of mourning a third party, the child, who could not possibly be created at that moment.

Without a knowledge of the fertility signs, it is easy to think one may not have any fertility at all. But after learning that the mucus makes a woman fertile for only a few days per cycle, couples begin to think in terms of how much combined fertility they may have. The focus changes powerfully from infertility to fertility, and from limitations to opportunities for conception.

Vaginal Infections

A vaginal infection, or vaginitis, is an itchy, painful infection of the vaginal area. Unpleasant-smelling discharges characteristically accompany vaginitis. Sometimes, invading organisms cause vaginal infections. In other cases, organisms normally found within the healthy vagina leap beyond their usual population limits.

A woman's own diet, level of stress, clothing, cleanliness, or other habits frequently create the conditions which favor vaginitis. Simple changes will usually improve her health.

In the meantime, home remedies for vaginitis are among the most effective and inexpensive treatments.

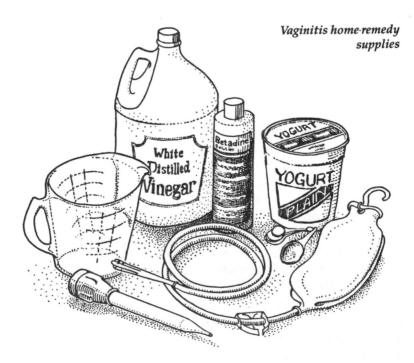

*Vaginitis home-remedy
supplies*

But please, don't try to cover up odors or symptoms with "feminine" douching or sprays. These products may only make matters worse. (In addition, douches and sprays may also hamper fertility by interfering with sperm movement.)

Mucus observations

Keep observing your mucus, but wipe more gently than usual. Even with the discharge from vaginitis, you will still be able to observe the changes from dry to fertile wetness and back to infertile dryness again. You might wish to use a temperature chart if your vulva is too irritated for good mucus observations.

To avoid transferring the infection back and forth between partners, avoid intercourse or carefully use a condom. Partners might refrain from intercourse anyway, because it can be too irritating or painful for the woman.

If they decide to use antibiotics for a vaginal infection, both partners should take a course of drugs, to avoid reinfecting each other. However, a woman may have chronic vaginitis caused by other medical conditions or drugs. In such a case, the man should not take antibiotics because the woman will continually reinfect him. After the woman's overall health improves, and she no longer takes the antibiotics which kill off her protective vaginal organisms, the couple may begin treatment together.

Self-help suggestions for discouraging vaginal infections

- Wear only clean dry all-cotton underwear.
- The vagina is self-cleansing. Douche with vinegar and water once a week if you feel you must douche.

- Do not douche or spray with "feminine hygiene" products. They disturb the natural organisms of the vagina and encourage infections.

- Exercise daily, to reduce stress and improve your health. Even a 10 minute daily walk is helpful.

- Practice stress management or relaxation exercises daily. Learn the techniques at a school evening course, from another knowledgeable person, or from a book or tape. Do more activities which you find enjoyable and relaxing.

- Eat unsweetened fresh fruit instead of sugary desserts and soda. Cut down on both refined sugar and artificial sweeteners.

- Avoid using birth control pills.

- Douche with yogurt and water, and eat yogurt while taking antibiotics, or Flagyl for vaginal infections. (Some women prefer using acidophilus lactobacillus culture rather than yogurt.)

- You may wish to cut down on your intake of antibiotics by avoiding commercially raised meat and poultry. (The animals are fed hormones and antibiotics which remain in their flesh.) Antibiotics kill many helpful vaginal organisms, allowing vaginal yeast to multiply wildly.

- Don't wear panty-shields every day, and change menstrual pads or tampons every three to four hours.

- Wipe downward, from front to back, when observing your mucus.

- Also wipe from front to back after defecating, and teach your daughters to do the same.

- Keep your genital area dry, and exposed to air whenever possible. Avoid wearing nylon hose, leotards, or a damp swimsuit for long periods of time.

- Some women get yeast infections when they are pregnant. After pregnancy, the infection should subside.

Common types of vaginal infections

Yeast (Candida albicans) formerly called Monilia

Symptoms. White "cottage cheesy" curd-like discharge, mushroomy, yeasty or baking soda odor. White patches on vagina, vulva or cervix. Painful intercourse, dry vagina, intense itching.

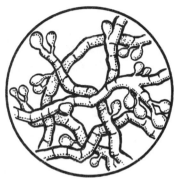

Yeast seen under microscope

Home remedies

Vinegar douche. Douche daily with 1-2 tablespoons of white vinegar in a quart of warm water, to restore acidity to the vagina.

Yogurt douche. Also douche with 4 tablespoons of plain unsweetened yogurt dissolved in a quart of water any time you feel itchy. You might douche 2-3 times a day for at least 3-4 days. The yogurt douche replaces helpful organisms in the vagina.

If infection continues, and you are neither pregnant, nor taking antibiotics or contraceptive pills, see your health care professional.

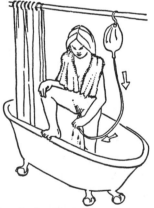

How to douche
Let fluids flow into the vagina very gently. Use a gravity douche bag or a gravy baster. Be sure your equipment is clean.

Trichomonas (Trich, pronounced "trick"), a parasite

Symptoms. Foul-smelling, gray or greenish yellow, thin or frothy discharge, may be streaked with blood or pus. Itching, soreness, burning of vagina or vulva. Frequent urination, bleeding, swollen pelvic glands. Vagina and cervix are mottled red (strawberry appearance).

Have the doctor confirm trich with a look under the microscope at a sample of the discharge in salt solution. One type of gonorrhea has similar symptoms and it is important to treat the infection you really have.[1]

Men's symptoms. Men may not have any symptoms, but can carry the organisms in their sexual organs. Men may have a slight discharge or tickling sensation of the penis. They should be treated to avoid giving the infection back to their partners.

Avoid intercourse, or use condoms until the infection is gone.

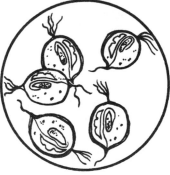

Trichomonas seen under the microscope

Home remedies

Betadine® douche. First douche with water and Betadine® solution, available at a drugstore. Use 1 tablespoon Betadine® in 1 quart of warm water, twice a day for 1 or 2 days maximum. This will kill most of the organisms in the vagina. *Do not douche with Betadine® while pregnant.*

Vinegar douche and yogurt douche. During the next week, douche daily, first with 1-2 tablespoons of white vinegar in 1 quart of water, then with 4 tablespoons plain, unsweetened yogurt in a quart of water.

Hemophilus, gardnerella, or other bacterial infection

Symptoms. Swollen, pus-covered vagina, itchy inflamed vulva, gray-white, yellow, or brown (bloody) foul-smelling discharge. The discharge may contain mucus, pus, blood, or bacteria.

The organisms can live in the man's urethra without any symptoms. Partners should avoid intercourse or use condoms until the infection is gone, to avoid reinfecting one another.

Causes. Wiping from back to front after defecating. Leaving menstrual pads or tampons in place too long; pads should ideally be changed every 3-4 hours. Wiping from back to front when observing the mucus; hands not clean when observing mucus.

Home remedies

Kill most of the bacteria with the Betadine® and water douche, as described under Trichomonas. Douche twice daily for one or two days. Then use the yogurt and water douche once or twice a day for two or three days to replace friendly organisms. If desired, douche daily for a week with vinegar and water.

Pinworms

Chronic vaginal irritation and infection may be caused by pinworms, especially if you live in a rural or poultry-producing location. If all the usual treatments have failed, have your doctor check for these parasites in the vagina.

Vaginal infections can impede sperm movement, and contribute to low fertility.

Finding A Teacher

Across the country and around the world there are literally thousands of teachers eager to help you learn to use your fertility signals.

Teachers may be listed in your White or Yellow Pages phone directory. Look under these headings:

- **Birth control:** ...Billings Ovulation Method...Fertility Awareness Method...Natural Family Planning...Ovulation Method...Rhythm Method (alternatives to)...Sympto-Thermal Method
- **Catholic Church**
- **Couple-to-Couple League**
- **Health Department or Division of Health Services,** state or county
- **Hospital,** education department or women's health center. Also check Catholic hospitals. (Note: many Catholic hospitals are named after saints.)
- **Planned Parenthood**
- **Women's Center,** community organized or at a university
- **Women's health clinic,** or women's health center at a hospital
- **University Health Center** on many campuses

When you talk to a teacher, find out...
- How long has he/she used the fertility signals?
- If the teacher's philosophical outlook on natural fertility control differs from yours, will you feel comfortable learning from her/him?
- Has the teacher been certified by one of the organizations listed below?

Ask if the instructor teaches the method you wish to learn

Ovulation, Mucus, or Original © Billings Ovulation Method. These methods use the mucus sign alone. While fertile, couples make love to become pregnant, or avoid pregnancy by refraining from intercourse. Also called OM.

Sympto-Thermal Method or Mucus/Temperature Method. STM uses mucus, plus temperature and/or cervical change. While fertile, couples make love to become pregnant, or avoid pregnancy by avoiding intercourse

Fertility Awareness Method. Using mucus, possibly temperature and/or cervical change. Flexible in working with clients who wish to continue using contraceptive barriers at times. (FAM is considered a barrier method since barrier use is included as an option. Teachers are careful to point out that FAM is less effective than the Ovulation or Sympto-Thermal methods for preventing pregnancy.)

Rhythm Method. Outdated and ineffective. Why guess when you might be fertile based on past cycles? Instead, learn how your mucus tells you whether you can or can't get pregnant, day by day.

You may find a teacher by contacting the organizations listed here. These listings are offered as a service and springboard to the reader. The author and publisher do not endorse or vouch for any of the teachers or organizations listed in this book - you must check them out for yourself.

By the way, *please be tolerant* of a teacher whose religious, or nonreligious, outlook differs from yours when she teaches about the fertility signals. After all, that dedicated person may be the only teacher in your area! Learn what you can, and practice it according to your own conscience.

In cases of confusing mucus patterns, or of low fertility, the very detailed Creighton Method can be of enormous help. For a teacher near you, contact: Creighton University, NFP Center, 6901 Mercy Rd., Omaha, NE 68106 USA. Phone (402) 390-9168

For Billings Method teachers phone NFP of Washington, D.C., (301) 530-9383.

If you cannot find a provider near you in this brief listing, you can get an accurate listing of NFP teachers who work under the auspices of the Catholic Church, plus some other teachers too, from:

Teresa Notare,
Diocesan Development Program for Natural Family Planning,
3211 4th St. NE, Washington, DC, 20017-1194. Phone (202) 541-3070

You may also call your local Catholic Diocesan Office, listed in the Yellow Pages.

Listed alphabetically by state:

Fertility Awareness
Sara Rose
P.O. Box 2802, Huntsville, AL 35804
English & Spanish

Cedars Sinai Medical Ctr.
8700 Beverly Blvd.
Los Angeles, CA 90048
Family Planning:
(310) 855-2000, 855-6411
English & Spanish

LA Regional Family Planning Council
3600 Wilshire Blvd., Ste. 600
Los Angeles, CA 90010
(213) 386-5614
English & Spanish

Center for Health Training
Marsha Gelt
2229 Lombard St.
San Francisco, CA 94123
(415) 563-0909
English & Spanish

WOOMB Bilingual/Bicultural
4422 Prospect
Yorbalinda, CA 92686
English & Spanish

Hannah Klaus, MD; NFP of Wash., DC
8514 Bradmoor
Bethesda, MD 20817
(301) 530-9383
Billings Ovulation Method, Teen Star Program, listings of Billings Method teachers.

Anne Lanctot - MD/DC Providers Assoc.
Box 29260, Washington, DC, 20017
(301) 853-4564
English & Spanish

Sharon Dausman - Illinois NFP Assoc.
155 E. Superior St.
Chicago, IL 60611
(312) 751-8339

St. Francis Regional Med. Ctr.
929 N. St. Francis
Wichita, KS 67214

Family of the Americas
1150 Lovers Lane
Mandeville, LA 70448
English & Spanish

KM Associates, Mary Shivanandan
PO Box 71041
Chevy Chase, MD 20813

Linda Nacleria
St. Mary's Women and Infant Ctr.
90 Cushing Ave.
Boston (Dorchester) MA 02125
(617) 436-8600, ext 474

Kay Ek, Dir, Office of NFP
316 N. 7th Ave.
St. Cloud, MN 56303
(320) 252-2100
(800) 864-6225

Aware Ctr. - St. Anthony's Hosp.
10010 Kennerly Rd.
St. Louis, MO 63128
(314) 525-1622

Fertility Awareness
P.O. Box 19875
St. Louis, MO 63144
(314) 968-2596

St. Johns Hosp. NFP Center
11700 Studt Ave
St. Louis, MO 63141
(314) 991-5766
Creighton Method, especially good for
confusing mucus patterns and low fertility.
Listing of teachers nationwide.

Kathy Rivet, Coord for NFP Office
Optimum Health Catholic Med. Ctr.
100 Mc. Gregor St., Manchestor, NH 03102
(603) 668-3545

NFP Center
St. Joseph's Hosp. NE Heights
PO Box 25555
Albuquerque, NM 87125
(505)888-7882

Family Life Info Ctr.
St. Peter's Hospital
315 S. Manning Blve.
Albany, NY 12208

The Fertility Awareness Ctr.
Barbara Feldman, Dir.
PO Box 2606, NY NY 10009
(212) 475-4490

Linda Bedo - NFP Office
Dicese of Raleigh
300 Cardinal Gibbons dr.
Raleigh, NC. 27606
(919) 821-0350

Couple-to-Couple League
Box 1184, Cincinnati, OH 45211
Spanish, French, Polish, Dutch.
Although their system is comlex, teachers
are listed in phone books of most cities.

Fertility Awareness Serices
Suzannah Cooper-Doyle
Box 986, Corvallis, OR 97339
(541) 753-8530

Rose Fuller- NW NFP Service
Providence Medical Center
4805 NE Glisan
Portland, OR 97213
English & Spanish

Rosemarie Kiesewetter
NFP of the Alleghenies
48 Seneca Ave, Altoona PA 16602
((814) 946-3544

Marge Harrigan, RN, BA
Supervisor and Educator of NFP
4639 Corona Dr. S., 13B
Corpus Christi, TX 78411
(512) 852-0222
English & Spanish

NFP Center
Sacred Heart Med. Ctr. Education
W. 101 8th Ave.
Spokane, WA 99204

Finding Out More

Fertility Awareness/Natural Family Planning Resource Directory
Fertility Awareness Services, $25.00
Edited by Suzannah Cooper-Doyle, © 1988 Small World Publications,
P.O. Box 986-W, Corvallis, OR 97339   *(541) 753-8530*

A comprehensive new review of fertility awareness and natural family planning books, fertility awareness method and NFP teaching aids, instructor's groups, women's health books, and health awareness information and groups. Resources on D.E.S., infertility, pregnancy, birth and parenting, and teen sex education are also reviewed in Cooper's flowing style. A must for every teacher, clinic, or individual who is interested in fertility awareness, natural family planning, or woman's health.

Also available: **Ovulation Method Instruction & Charting Booklet, $6.50; A Fertility Awareness Self-Instruction Course, $45; Fertility Factsheets; Individual Mucus/BBT charts, full page, .25 each.** Send $.50 plus self-addressed, stamped envelope for descriptive list.

KM Associates

P.O. Box 71041, Chevy Chase, MD 20813-1041, phone (301) 652-4534
Books, including *Challenge to Love,* and information sheets focusing on the relationship of the couple who uses natural family planning. To receive *KM Kaleidoscope,* an ongoing information sheet highlighting publicity resources (including mailing lists) for natural family planning groups, send $2.00 plus self-addressed stamped envelope.

Boston Women's Health Book Collective *47 Nichols Ave.* *Watertown, MA 02172*	*Vancouver Women's Health Collective* *Suite 213* *1675 W. 8th Ave.* *Vancouver, BC* *Canada V6J-1V2* *phone (604)-736-4234* *(604)-736-5262*

These groups carry outstanding selections of women's health and fertility awareness books. Send $.25 and a self-addressed stamped envelope for a price-list.

For Further Reading

Aguilar, Nona. *The New No-Pill, No-Risk Birth Control,* Rawson Associates, New York, 1986.

Billings, Evelyn; Billings, John; Catarinich, M. *Atlas of the Ovulation Method,* Ovulation Method Research & Reference Center of Australia, 27 Alexandra Pde., North Fitzroy, Victoria, 3068, Australia, ©1973-1989. Breastfeeding section answers all questions. Book is essential for all users/teachers of natural methods.

Billings, Dr. Evelyn, & Westmore, Ann. *The Billings Method: Controlling Fertility Without Drugs or Devices,* Random House, New York, 1980. Ballantine paperback. Comprehensive, easy to understand, one of best books on the topic. Dr. John Billings and Dr. Evelyn Billings developed the modern © Billings Ovulation Method. $8.95

Boston Women's Health Book Collective. *The New Our Bodies, Ourselves.* Simon & Schuster, 1984. $14.95. Learn about all aspects of how your body works and what to do to take care of it yourself.

Canfield, Jack, and Noble, Georgia. *Living and Loving: Couples Seminar, and Self Esteem Seminars Exercises and Tapes.* Self Esteem Seminars, 17156 Palisades Circle, Pacific Palisades, CA 90272. Enjoyable, practical; help you create more loving relationships with yourself and others.

Cooper-Doyle, Suzannah. Indispensable books for class or home.
A Fertility Awareness and Natural Family Planning Resource Directory copyright 1988; $25.00
Ovulation Method 3-Year Charting Booklet (with directions), $6.50
Fertility Awareness Self-Instruction Course, $45.00
Fertility Factsheets
Individual Mucus/BBT charts, full page, .25 each
Fertility Awareness Services, P.O. Box 986-W, Corvallis, OR 97339

Hilgers, Dr. Thomas W., and others, including Daly, K.Diane; Hilgers, Susan K.; and Prebil, Ann M. Works are available from *Pope Paul VI Institute, 6901 Mercy Road, Omaha, Nebraska, 68106*
Picture Dictionary of the Ovulation Method. Excellent photographs of the types of cervical mucus. A very useful teaching aid.
Articles and papers (Interesting despite very small sample groups):
The Peak Symptom and Estimated Time of Ovulation, Obstetrics & Gynecology, Vol. 52, November 1978.
The Ovulation Method — Vulvar Observations as an Index of Fertility/Infertility, Obstetrics & Gynecology, Vol. 53, No. 1, January 1979.
Natural Family Planning II. Basal Body Temperature and Estimated Time of Ovulation, Obstetrics & Gynecology, Vol. 55, No. 3, March 1980.
Natural Family Planning IV. The Identification of Postovulatory Infertility, Obstetrics and Gynecology, Vol. 58, No. 3, September 1981.

Federation of Feminist Women's Health Centers. *A New View of a Woman's Body.* Simon and Schuster, New York, 1981. Beautifully illustrated, easy to read guide to the woman's body and health care, emphasizing self-help, no-holds-barred information, and women helping each other.

Kass-Annese, Barbara, and Danzer, Hal, M.D. *The Fertility Awareness Workbook.* *Printed Matter, Inc., P.O. Box 15246, Atlanta, GA 30333. $7.95.* Large format, well-suited for class or home.

Lacey, Louise. *Lunaception. McCann & Geoghegan, 1974.* Currently out of print, but authorized photocopied copies are available for $11 from *Louise Lacey, P.O. Box 489, Berkely, CA 94701.* How to regulate your cycles with light, why light regulation works, and how Ms. Lacey found out.

Nofziger, Margaret. *A Cooperative Method of Natural Birth Control. The Book Publishing Company, Summertown, Tennessee, USA 38483.* © 1974. Lighthearted and easy to use, $7.00.

Shettles, Dr. Landrum B., and Rorvik, David M. *Choose Your Baby's Sex: the One Sex Selection Method That Works. Dodd, Mead & Company, New York, 1977.* Explains the connection between sex selection and the time of ovulation. Does not mention cervical mucus.

Shivanandan, Mary. *Challenge to Love. KM Associates, Associates, P.O. Box 71041, Chevy Chase, Maryland 20813-1041. $5.95,* quantity discounts. Explores the many facets of periodic abstinence, from resentment and resistance, to transcendence and unity with one's partner and God. Includes examples of users from a wide variety of religious and cultural groups.

Wilson, Mercedes. *The Ovulation Method of Birth Regulation, The Latest Advances for Achieving or Postponing Pregnancy — Naturally. Van Nostrand Reinhold Company, 1980. Order from Family of the Americas Foundation, P.O. Box 219, Mandeville, LA 70448. (504) 626-7724.* Highlights ovulation method programs in developing countries. Describes user education levels, details many effectiveness studies. Demonstrates that women of any educational and cultural background can successfully use and teach the ovulation method.

Vollman, R. F. *The Menstrual Cycle. W. B. Saunders Co., Philadelphia, 1977, out of print (obtain at a medical school library).* Thorough study and analysis of 20,000 temperature charts from 656 women during 30 years.

References

(In addition to the authors referred to below, many others have delved into the science of the fertility signals. Space does not permit a complete listing, but among the early researchers are J. Brown, H. Burger, and E. Odeblad, on mucus, and J. Roetzer, on temperature.)

YOUR FERTILITY SIGNALS, THE FACTS, pp. 1-11
1. E. L. Billings, A. Westmore, *The Billings Method*, Random House, New York, 1980, p. 200. *"The Peak mucus signal, as judged by women themselves, occurs on the average 0.6 (fourteen hours) before ovulation. In about 85 per cent of women, the Peak occurs within a day of ovulation and in 95 per cent, within two days."*
2. ibid.
3. T. W. Hilgers, G. E. Abraham, D. Cavanaugh, *The Peak Symptom and Estimated Time of Ovulation*, Obstetrics and Gynecology, Vol. 52, No. 5, Nov. 1978, p. 575. *"In 65 cycles of 75 studied in 24 patients, there was hormonal confirmation of ovulation . . . In the 65 normal cycles, 64 exhibited a Peak symptom. In those cycles, ovulation was estimated to occur from 3 days before to 3 days after the Peak symptom with a mean of .31 days before the Peak symptom. In 95.4% of these cycles, ovulation was estimated to occur from 2 days before to 2 days after the Peak symptom."*
4. E. L. Billings, op. cit. p. 30.
5. E. L. Billings, op. cit. p. 12.
6. S. Cooper, *Infertility Troubleshooting*, Small World Publications, Corvallis Oregon, 1985.

ADDED DIMENSIONS, pp. 12-15
1. E. L. Billings, op. cit., p. 20. *"The laboratory studies of the mucus, the laparoscopic data, the hormonal assays and the infertility research, have all provided confirmatory evidence that a woman's own awareness provides an extremely accurate guide to her state of fertility."*
   and, E. L. Billings, op. cit., pp. 198-199. *"Professor James Brown . . . [was] involved helping sub-fertile couples achieve a pregnancy . . . by timing intercourse with laboratory measurements of the peak level of the hormone oestrogen. This approach proved relatively successful, but [he] later confirmed that womens' own awareness of their cervical mucus could indicate ovulation even more accurately than oestrogen measurements."*
2. E. L. Billings, op. cit., p. 217-219. The World Health Organization conducted a study in 1976-1978, of 875 women in New Zealand, Ireland, India, the Philippines, and El Salvador. Results indicated that: *"The method failure rate of this and similar studies is between 1% and 3% . . . (The method-related pregnancy rate was 0.9% for the three cycles of observations during the teaching phase, a period too short to make reliable judgments about overall method effectiveness. The teaching related pregnancy rate [due to poor or incorrect instruction] was 5.3%. Conscious departure from the method accounted for 12.9% and unexplained was 0.9%.)* <u>*The vast majority of these pregnancies followed intercourse during the phase of recognized fertility.)*</u>*"* (Emphasis added.)

LEARNING, pp. 16-19
1. E. L. Billings, op. cit., p. 218. *"At least 90% of women can produce a recognisable chart of their fertility after one teaching session. By the third teaching session, at least 94% can recognise such a pattern."*

YOUR MUCUS SIGNAL, THE OVULATION METHOD, pp. 20-45
1. E. L. Billings, op. cit., T. W. Hilgers, et. al., op. cit.

YOUR TEMPERATURE SIGNAL, pp. 46-55
1. R. F. Vollman, *The Menstrual Cycle*, W. B. Saunders Co., Philadelphia, 1977. After studying 20,672 menstrual cycles with BBT records, he concluded: *"The day-to-day succession of the basal body temperatures shows all possible variations within the same woman and between different women. It is therefore, difficult to define a practical number of patterns without producing abstract and potentially distorted plots. The daily fluctuations of the BBT are peculiar to the individual woman; in fact, they are personally characteristic."*

ENERGY, MOODS, AND FERTILITY CHANGES, pp. 56-59
1. R. Rosenthal, electrologist, personal observation to author.
2. L. Robertson, C. Flinders, B. Godfrey, *Laurel's Kitchen, a Handbook for Vegetarian Cookery and Nutrition*, Bantam Books, 13th printing, April 1982, p. 473.
3. L. Robertson, et. al., op. cit., p. 492.
4. L. Robertson, et. al., op. cit., p. 498.

PRACTICAL STRATEGIES, pp. 60-69
1. G. Noble, J. Canfield, an exercise from the *Relationship Seminar*, April 1986, Self Esteem Seminars, Pacific Palisades, California.
2. G. Noble, J. Canfield, op. cit.
3. Courtesy of S. Cooper, from her Fertility Awareness Library, Corvallis, Oregon.
4. Courtesy of S. Cooper, collected from various sources.

AFTER THE PILL, pp. 80-83
1. J. Willis, *'The Pill' May Not Mix Well With Other Drugs*, FDA Consumer, March 1987, p. 27.
2. E. L. Billings, op. cit., p. 169.
3. J. Willis, op. cit., p. 27.
4. D. Feingold, *NEWS: Antibiotic Birth Control Interactions*, OB-GYN News, Vol. 21, No. 21.
5. J. Willis, op. cit., p. 26-28.

REGULATING CYCLES WITH LIGHT, pp. 84-85
(*Also see:* J. de Felice, *The Effects of Light on Cervical Mucus Patterns*, Spokan⁻ 'Nashington)
1. L. Lacey, *Lunaception, A Feminine Odyssey into Fertility and Contraception*, 1975, p. 117.
2. Dewan, and J. Rock, *Photic effects upon the human menstrual cycle: statistical evidence*, John Rock Institute, Boston. Described by L. Lacey, *Lunaception* article, CoEvolution Quarterly, Winter Solstice, 1974, p. 84. *"Several possible sequences of three [nights of light] were tried, but none had any effect on ovulation at all—but one. When the light burned on the 14th, 15th, and 16th days . . . previously irregular, infertile women were able to entrain their ovulation cycles into a regular 29-day rhythm, ovulating predictably on the 14th or 15th day."*
3. L. Lacey, op. cit., pp. 101-102.
4. Midrashic tradition related by Rabbi S. Talve, St. Louis, Mo.

CHOOSING YOUR BABY'S SEX, pp. 86-89
1. Dr. (Sr.) Leonie McSweeney, Report to VIth International Institute of the Ovulation Method, Los Angeles, California, referred to by E.L. Billings, op. cit., p. 70.
2. L. Shettles, D. Rorvik, *Choose Your Baby's Sex: the One Sex Selection Method That Works*, Dodd, Mead, & Co., N.Y., 1977.
3. ibid.

MENOPAUSE, THE NATURAL WAY, pp. 90-93
1. E. L. Billings, op. cit., p. 215.

HORMONES TRIGGER THE FERTILITY SIGNALS, pp. 94-101
1. E. L. Billings, op. cit., page 200
   T. W. Hilgers, et. al., op. cit.

INFERTILITY SELF-HELP, pp. 102-129
1. S. Cooper and B. Feldman, fertility awareness instructors. Their experience with many sub-fertile clients has shown this to be an effective approach.
2. M. Perloe, *Miracle Babies*, Penguin Books, N.Y., 1987, p. 38. However, a physician *may* be board certified in the reproductive endocrinology and infertility subspecialty.
3. J. A. McCoshen, *The role of cervical mucus production in reproduction*, Contemporary OB/GYN, May 1987, p. 100. The article explains an array of factors involved in sperm/mucus interactions, and specifically questions whether sperm antibodies are the problem they are thought to be. *"In one couple, both partners had the highest titers of sperm antibodies ever encountered in our laboratory [for sperm, cervical mucus and seminal fluid]. Nevertheless, the woman eventually became pregnant without treatment."*
4. T. W. Hilgers, K. D. Daly, S. K. Hilgers, A. M. Prebil, *The Ovulation Method of Natural Family Planning, a Standardized Case Management Approach to Teaching, Book One*, Creighton University N.F.P. Education and Research Center, Omaha, Nebraska, 1982, p. 56.
5. E. L. Billings, op. cit., p. 151.
6. M. McKay, lecture at Ovulation Method Teachers Association Conference, 1987.
7. ibid.
8. G. W. Bates, quoted by J. Graham and S. Ince, *When Thin is Not In*, Self Magazine, Nov. 1988, p. 197.
9. L. Lacey, op. cit.; also S. Cooper and B. Feldman, fertility awareness teachers, experiences with clients.
10. M. Perloe, op. cit., p. 133.
11. J. Canfield, G. Noble, *Self Esteem Seminars*, Pacific Palisades, California.

VAGINAL INFECTIONS, pp. 130-135
1. S. Kramer, *Vaginal Infections*, NFP Advocate.

Glossary

anovulatory cycle Cycle in which no egg is released.

barrier, or barrier method Condom, diaphragm, cervical cap, or other device, usually used with spermicides, to prevent sperm from entering the cervix.

basal body temperature A person's temperature when first awakening after at least three to four hours of sleep.

BBT Basal body temperature.

BBT method Using awareness of the temperature signal to identify when ovulation is over and the woman is no longer fertile.

cephalad change Using the changes in cervical shape and position for fertility awareness.

cervical crypts Tiny folds within the cervix that make cervical mucus and shelter a man's sperm cells during the fertile phase.

cervical mucus Wet, smooth, slippery and/or stretchy substance which the cervix secretes in response to the estrogen from ripening eggs. Cervical mucus signals a woman's fertility. The mucus also nourishes and protects a man's sperm cells until ovulation, and permits them to swim through the woman's cervix.

cervix The lower part of the uterus which extends into the vagina. The cervix produces fertile-type cervical mucus.

cilia Tiny hairlike structures lining the fallopian tubes. The cilia help propel the egg toward the uterus.

conceive To become pregnant.

conception The union of the woman's egg cell with the man's sperm cell.

condom A sheath of plastic or animal membrane placed over the penis to catch seminal fluid and keep sperm from entering the vagina. The condom can also prevent certain bacteria and infections from being passed between partners.

corpus luteum After ovulation, the follicle which had surrounded the ripening egg becomes the corpus luteum. The corpus luteum secretes progesterone hormone which is needed to maintain both the enriched uterine lining, and pregnancy itself.

diaphragm A round plastic barrier, spread with spermicidal cream or jelly and placed within the vagina to prevent sperm cells from entering the cervix.

douche Washing the vagina with water or another solution. Ordinarily, douching is unnecessary because the vagina is self-cleansing. Douching is mainly useful for treating vaginal infections.

dry day When there is no fertile mucus at any time throughout the day or evening.

early withdrawal Removing the penis from the vagina before the man ejaculates. Early withdrawal can cause pregnancy during the fertile phase because the man can have a drop of sperm-filled fluid at the opening of his penis long before ejaculating. Also known as "withdrawal," "coitus interruptus," or "taking it out."

egg The woman's cell which, after union with the man's sperm, can become a new baby.

ejaculation Release of semen from the penis, usually after physical and/or emotional stimulation.

endometrium Inner lining of the uterus. The endometrium grows thicker and blood-enriched in response to estrogen, and maintains its thickness in response to progesterone. Menstruation is the shedding of the endometrium.

estrogen The female hormone which is secreted by the follicle around the ripening egg in the ovary. Estrogen causes the uterine lining to become thick and blood-enriched, keeps the BBT low, makes the cervix soft, open and high, and triggers ovulation. Fat cells convert adrenal androgens to estrogen and help maintain the estrogen level after menopause.

fallopian tubes Tubes through which the egg travels to the uterus.

fertile time Beginning when the woman has fertile cervical mucus, and ending on the evening of the fourth dry (non-mucus) day in a row after the mucus ends.

fertile mucus Cervical mucus.

fertility awareness Being able to identify the fertile and infertile phases using the natural fertility signals.

fertility awareness method Using fertility awareness to identify the woman's fertile and infertile phases. Having intercourse while fertile to become pregnant, and avoiding intercourse or using barrier methods while fertile to prevent pregnancy.

fertilization The fusion of sperm and egg.

follicle Surrounds the ripening egg in the ovary and produces the hormone estrogen.

follicle stimulating hormone (FSH) A pituitary hormone that causes egg development.

genital-to-genital contact Any touching of penis to vagina, penis to vulva, or semen to fertile mucus.

hormone A chemical messenger within the body.

hypothalamus Gland in the brain which helps control the hormonal events leading to ovulation.

implantation When the fertilized egg buries itself in the blood-enriched uterine lining.

intercourse Sexual contact with the penis inside the vagina. Also called sexual intercourse or making love.

luteinizing hormone A pituitary hormone which prompts the follicle to burst through the side of the ovary, releasing the egg.

making love Intercourse.

menopause The time in a woman's life when she no longer menstruates and is not fertile anymore.

menstruation Shedding of the blood-enriched uterine lining, usually about two weeks after ovulation (if the woman did not become pregnant in that cycle).

mucus, cervical or fertile Cervical mucus.

ovary One of two small female organs which contain immature and ripening eggs.

ovulation Release of one or more ripe eggs from the ovary.

ovulation method Using awareness of the mucus signal to identify infertile and fertile phases. Having intercourse while fertile, to become pregnant, or avoiding intercourse while fertile to avoid pregnancy.

Peak day Last day of any wet, smooth, slippery and/or stretchy cervical mucus, or non-menstrual spotting.

penis External male organ of reproduction, urination and sexual response. Semen and sperm cells are ejaculated through the urinary opening at the tip of the penis.

pituitary gland Gland within the brain which secretes hormones that control the timing of ovulation.

progesterone Hormone secreted by the corpus luteum. After ovulation, progesterone raises the woman's BBT and maintains both the blood-enriched uterine lining and pregnancy.

prolactin A hormone which stimulates milk production during breast-feeding and inhibits ovulation.

rhythm method Outdated way of guessing when a woman is fertile based on her previous cycle lengths and temperature charts.

semen Whitish fluid normally containing sperm cells, ejaculated from the man's penis.

sperm cells The tiny cells from a man which, after uniting with a woman's egg, can grow into a new individual.

spermicide Jelly, cream, foam, suppositories, or other substances which are meant to damage or kill sperm cells in order to prevent pregnancy.

sympto-thermal method Using awareness of mucus, temperature, and/or cervical change signals to identify the fertile and infertile phases. Having intercourse while fertile to become pregnant, or refraining from intercourse when fertile, to avoid pregnancy.

testes (testicles) Two round external male organs which produce sperm cells and some male hormones.

uterine lining Endometrium.

uterus (womb) A muscular, hollow female organ of reproduction and sexual response. The lining of the uterus grows and then is shed as the menstrual flow during each cycle. During pregnancy, the fetus grows inside the uterus.

vagina (birth canal) An elastic canal between the cervix and the vulva. Wet, slippery mucus slides down the tightly closed walls of the vagina to the vaginal opening.

vulva External opening of the vagina.

withdrawal Early withdrawal.

Index

| | | | | | | | Month | Year |

TEMPERATURE
(Yours may be lower or higher)

DAY OF CYCLE / WEEK DAY / DATE / SEX / SYMBOL

MUCUS DESCRIPTION

97   97.5   98   98.5   99

Day
1
2
3
4
5
6
7
8
9
10
11
12
13
14
15
16
17
18
19
20
21
22
23
24
25
26
27
28
29
30
31
32
33
34
35
36
37
38
39
40

● Menstruation   ❀ Spotting
□ Dry   ■ Wet, slippery or stretchy
1,2,3,4—Infertile the evening of the fourth dry day in a row
after the last bit of mucus or non-menstrual spotting

THINK—*Wet or dry?*
WIPE—*Dry? Wet, smooth or slippery?*
LOOK—*Creamy, stretchy, nothing? If you
feel or see mucus you are fertile*

Month   Year

TEMPERATURE
(Yours may be lower or higher)

DAY OF CYCLE / WEEK DAY / DATE / SEX / SYMBOL

MUCUS DESCRIPTION

97   97.5   98   98.5   99

1	
2	
3	
4	
5	
6	
7	
8	
9	
10	
11	
12	
13	
14	
15	
16	
17	
18	
19	
20	
21	
22	
23	
24	
25	
26	
27	
28	
29	
30	
31	
32	
33	
34	
35	
36	
37	
38	
39	
40	

● Menstruation   ⋰ Spotting
□ Dry   ■ Wet, slippery or stretchy
1,2,3,4—Infertile the evening of the fourth dry day in a row
         after the last bit of mucus or non-menstrual spotting

THINK—*Wet or dry?*
WIPE—*Dry? Wet, smooth or slippery?*
LOOK—*Creamy, stretchy, nothing? If you
       feel or see mucus you are fertile*

TEMPERATURE
(Yours may be lower or higher)

DAY OF CYCLE	WEEK DAY	DATE	SEX	SYMBOL	MUCUS DESCRIPTION	97	97.5	98	98.5	99
1										
2										
3										
4										
5										
6										
7										
8										
9										
10										
11										
12										
13										
14										
15										
16										
17										
18										
19										
20										
21										
22										
23										
24										
25										
26										
27										
28										
29										
30										
31										
32										
33										
34										
35										
36										
37										
38										
39										
40										

● Menstruation   •• Spotting
□ Dry   ■ Wet, slippery or stretchy
1,2,3,4—Infertile the evening of the fourth dry day in a row
after the last bit of mucus or non-menstrual spotting

THINK—*Wet or dry?*
WIPE—*Dry? Wet, smooth or slippery?*
LOOK—*Creamy, stretchy, nothing? If you
feel or see mucus you are fertile*

TEMPERATURE
(Yours may be lower or higher)

DAY OF CYCLE / WEEK DAY / DATE / SEX / SYMBOL

MUCUS DESCRIPTION   97   97.5   98   98.5   99

1	
2	
3	
4	
5	
6	
7	
8	
9	
10	
11	
12	
13	
14	
15	
16	
17	
18	
19	
20	
21	
22	
23	
24	
25	
26	
27	
28	
29	
30	
31	
32	
33	
34	
35	
36	
37	
38	
39	
40	

● Menstruation   ⣰ Spotting

☐ Dry   ■ Wet, slippery or stretchy

1,2,3,4—Infertile the evening of the fourth dry day in a row
after the last bit of mucus or non-menstrual spotting

THINK—*Wet or dry?*
WIPE—*Dry? Wet, smooth or slippery?*
LOOK—*Creamy, stretchy, nothing? If you
feel or see mucus you are fertile*

Help Others Find This Book

Many other women (and men) in your area would like to learn fertility awareness, but can't find good directions. Your enthusiasm can help them discover this book. Show a copy to your
> book seller,
>> librarian,
>>> natural food store manager,
>>>> midwife, nurse & doctor
>>>> women's center,
>>>>> family planning center,
>>>>>> childbirth educator
>>>>>>> La Leche League instructor

Encourage them to stock *YOUR FERTILITY SIGNALS.* Then other women will be able to find copies of the book so they can use and enjoy natural fertility control.

By the way, *please* tell retailers and librarians that the following distributors, *plus dozens* of others, can supply *YOUR FERTILITY SIGNALS:*

RETAIL & LIBRARY WHOLESALERS
Baker & Taylor
Bookpeople (English & Spanish)
Brodart
Downtown Book Center, Miami
Emery-Pratt
Ingram (English & Spanish)
Koen (English & Spanish)
Midwest Library Services
Moving Books
New Leaf
Nutri-Books (Eng. & Sp.)
Pacific Pipeline
Quality Books

If your bookstore does not carry **YOUR FERTILITY SIGNALS,**
you can easily order it from Smooth Stone Press,
in English, Spanish, German, or Chinese.

_____One copy, $13.95 + $2.00 postage = $15.95

_____Five copies, $11.95 each, + $5.25 postage = $60

_____Ten copies, $9.95 each, + $6.50 postage = $105

Please write for quantity discounts.
Missouri residents add 6% sales tax.

Name_____

Street _____

City_____State/Zip_____

Phone(____)_____

How did you find out about this book?_____

_____

To receive your books, simply
fill out coupon & send with check or money order to:

SMOOTH STONE PRESS
PO Box 19875, St. Louis, Missouri, USA 63144

Please indicate languages desired if other than English.
Shipping overseas, postage is $8.00 for first book, $2.00 each
additional book, USA funds only. Available directly from
stores in South & Central America (Spanish - published by
norma), Europe (German - published by Martin Ehrenwirth)
and Taiwan (Chinese - published by Morning Star, Tai Yea).

About the author and illustrator

MERRYL WINSTEIN holds a Bachelor of Fine Arts with a Minor in Biology from Washington University in St. Louis. She first learned about the fertility signals by reading and taking a natural family planning class at a hospital. Since then, as a teacher, she has revealed the simple secrets of the fertility signals to hundreds of women across the nation.

Ms. Winstein loves to get mail from readers, and will answer all letters accompanied by a self-addressed, stamped envelope.